The Source for School-Age Stuttering

Nina A. Reardon

J. Scott Yaruss

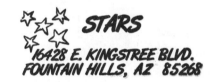

STARS
16428 E. KINGSTREE BLVD.
FOUNTAIN HILLS, AZ 85268

Age Level: 7 thru 18
Grades: 1 thru 12

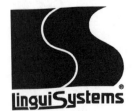

LinguiSystems, Inc.
3100 4th Avenue
East Moline, IL 61244-9700
1-800 PRO IDEA
1-800-776-4332

FAX: 1-800-577-4555
E-mail: service@linguisystems.com
Web: www.linguisystems.com
TDD: 1-800-933-8331
(for those with hearing impairments)

ISBN 0-7606-0448-7

About the Authors

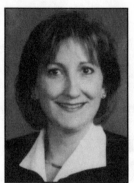

Nina A. Reardon, M.S. CCC-SLP, is a speech-language pathologist providing services to several rural school districts in Illinois. She also specializes in providing stuttering therapy services to children and adolescents in private practice. Nina has published materials for both the Stuttering Foundation of America and the National Stuttering Association (NSA). She is a member of the American Speech-Language and Hearing Association Division #4's Task Force for Insurance Reimbursement, and is a member of the Board of Directors of the NSA where she serves on the Executive Committee and as the Chairperson of NSA's National Family Programs. Nina presents interactive workshops on practical assessment and treatment strategies for preschool and school-age children who stutter.

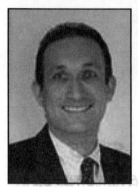

J. Scott Yaruss, Ph.D., CCC-SLP, is an Associate Professor at the University of Pittsburgh, the Co-Director of the Stuttering Center of Western Pennsylvania, and a Clinical Research Consultant at Children's Hospital of Pittsburgh. Scott serves on the Board of Directors for the NSA and on the Steering Committee of the Special Interest Division for Fluency and Fluency Disorders of the American Speech-Language-Hearing Association. Scott's research, which has received funding from the National Institutes of Health, focuses on the development of stuttering in young children as well as on the documentation of treatment outcomes in adults who stutter. Scott is a frequent presenter of continuing education presentations and workshops on treatment strategies for preschoolers and school-age children who stutter, as well as on practical counseling techniques for SLPs.

Dedications

Dedicated to my co-author, J. Scott Yaruss, whose unconditional passion for improving the lives of people who stutter inspire all those who are lucky enough to know you. Thank you, Scotch, for your wisdom, support, and above all, your friendship. Without these blessings, neither this book nor this past year of my own journey could have been realized. — NAR

Dedicated to the memory of Melvin P. Yaruss, a loving friend and grandfather who demonstrated by his life that stuttering does not have to hold you back or define who you are. Thank you for providing such a wonderful example. — JSY

Acknowledgments

We would like to express our sincere appreciation and admiration for our many colleagues and friends who have dedicated their lives to helping people who stutter. We have been inspired and encouraged by your example. So many of the ideas expressed in this book are drawn from your work, and we are grateful for the model you have provided. We are particularly grateful for the many helpful comments provided by Craig Coleman, Patti Bohlman, Barbara Weber, Lee Reeves, Bill Murphy, Steven B. Hood, and Bob Quesal. We would also like to thank the many children and families who have allowed us into their lives so we could join them on their "journey" for a time. We have been inspired by you, too, and we are grateful for the trust you placed in us. Finally, to our families, we express our deepest debt of gratitude for your patience, encouragement, and constant support. We could not have done any of this without you.*

Table of Contents

4

Who Should Read This Book?

The Source for School-Age Stuttering is written for speech-language pathologists (SLPs) who work with school-age children who stutter. We know that many clinicians have questions about preschool children who stutter and we recognize that there is a need for information about topics such as early intervention and therapy approaches for preschoolers who stutter and their families. We also know, however, that preschool stuttering therapy and school-age stuttering therapy are *very different* from one another. These differences influence not only the strategies clinicians use in therapy, but also the overall goals of intervention. Because of the fundamental differences between preschool and school-age stuttering, we cannot adequately address both age groups within one book. Therefore, this book is focused solely on the needs of clinicians working with school-age children who stutter.

Our goal is to discuss the entire stuttering disorder—not just the observable stuttering behaviors that are so often the focus of treatment. To most effectively help children who stutter, we must also examine the overall impact that the stuttering behaviors can have on the child's life. We will consider children's speech not only at school, but in *all* communicative environments and in *all* stages of their development. We will look at how children who stutter view themselves as communicators, and how this affects their interactions with other people. We will analyze all phases of the therapeutic process from assessment and diagnosis through treatment, and we will highlight the clinical skills that clinicians need to develop in order to foster long-term success for their students. Throughout this process, we will emphasize the necessity of tailoring treatment to the individual needs of each child and helping each child become the most effective communicator he or she can be.

How Is This Book Organized?

In *The Source for School-Age Stuttering*, we have attempted to address a wide variety of topics, from the basis of what stuttering is to more advanced discussions of how to develop the clinical skills you will need to prepare effective therapy plans. So whether you are a beginner or a veteran clinician, we hope that you will find tips for expanding your skills and validation for your existing skills.

Most books on stuttering include basic information about the background and theory of the disorder followed by discussions of assessment and treatment strategies. This necessary information is also presented in this book, though we have organized the information within the framework of the questions that frequently arise during the course of stuttering therapy. Our goal is to take you on a journey to increase your understanding of stuttering, while at the same time helping you develop the strategies and clinical skills you need to help children who stutter. We want you to increase your comfort with stuttering so you will be fully available to help your students with all aspects of this disorder.

The most important thing to know about the organization of this book is that within these pages, you will NOT find a programmed approach to stuttering therapy. The *Source for School-Age Stuttering* provides skills, strategies, and support as you seek to expand your knowledge and confidence in clinical problem solving for stuttering therapy. We recognize that many of you are looking for a guide to tell you "what to do." We believe that by developing a thorough understanding of the rationale for school-age stuttering therapy, you will feel more confident knowing what to do on your own, and you will feel less of a need for such a guide. Thus, our goal in writing this book is to help you develop the background and the skills you need to become an effective stuttering therapist without the need for a step-by-step guide.

How Can I Get More Comfortable with Stuttering?

The field of speech-language pathology is deeply rooted in the study of stuttering. In fact, the very first SLPs were scientists working to understand this disorder. For decades, clinicians and researchers have proposed numerous ideas about the cause of stuttering and about the best way to treat people who stutter. The rich history of theory and thought has resulted in a large body of literature about the nature and treatment of stuttering. Unfortunately, it has also had the unintended consequence of alienating many excellent clinicians who may feel (or who may have been told) that stuttering is "too complicated" and "too difficult" for them to treat. In fact, the majority of SLPs report that they are not comfortable with their abilities to work with children who stutter. They either feel that their training was inadequate or they feel that they do not see enough children who stutter to maintain their competence in this area.

One of our main goals in writing *The Source for School-Age Stuttering* is to help practicing clinicians recognize their strengths for working with children who stutter. We firmly believe that stuttering can be successfully treated in a variety of settings, including the schools. We want those of you who read this book to realize that you already possess many of the skills you need to successfully treat children who stutter. For example, clinicians commonly use hierarchies to introduce new concepts in therapy for many disorders. When working with children with speech sound disorders, we may use hierarchies to introduce target sounds in increasingly complex contexts (e.g., syllable, word, phrase). When working with children with language disorders, we may use hierarchies to introduce sentence structures with increasing complexity or narratives with increasing elaboration. In the same way, you can use hierarchies with children who stutter to gradually introduce new skills for managing stuttering in different contexts. Throughout this book, we will highlight many ways you can draw upon your existing clinical knowledge to enhance your stuttering therapy.

In writing this book, we have recalled many of the questions and comments we have heard from clinicians who have, at times, struggled with their comfort levels when working with people who stutter. Many of the chapter headings directly reflect the frustration and uncertainty we heard from parents and SLPs who wanted to help children who stutter but didn't know how. Indeed, we have often felt these same concerns. As our own understanding of the disorder has grown, however, we have come to realize that these frustrations can be overcome and that we *can* provide excellent service for people who stutter.

Although the headings sometimes reflect frustration, the text within the chapters reflects the positive opportunities that are available to clinicians working with children who stutter. We know from personal experience that clinicians can increase their confidence in their clinical skills. This increased confidence translates directly into greater comfort with stuttering and, ultimately, to more effective treatment for children who stutter. Before you can reach this point, however, you must face any fears you may have about your understanding of stuttering and your abilities to successfully assess and treat children who stutter. This is where we will begin our journey.

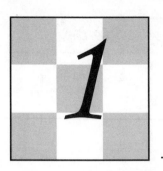

Help! This Child Stutters

It is widely recognized that stuttering is not the "favorite" disorder area for many speech-language pathologists (SLPs) to work with (St. Louis & Durrenberger 1993). We have talked to countless clinicians who have expressed frustration, fear, anxiety, or even disappointment when they learn that they have a child who stutters on their caseload. In this book, our goal is to help you feel more comfortable with stuttering—and with your clinical skills for treating stuttering—so you will not experience these negative reactions when working with children who stutter.

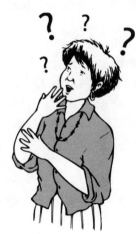

SLPs receive new students on their caseloads in a number of ways. Many times, we "inherit" a child from another clinician who worked with the child before. Other times, a parent or teacher may ask us to "take a quick look" at a child "just to see how his speech is doing." In either case, we need to determine for ourselves whether the child is stuttering, whether the child needs treatment, and if so, what the nature of that treatment should be. As a result, one of the first questions we tend to ask ourselves is "does this child really stutter?"

Does This Child Stutter?

Although this may seem like a straightforward question, it is not always easy to answer. This is because stuttering is expressed in so many ways. Some children stutter with repetitions but have very little physical tension or struggle. Others stutter with more physical tension or with prolongations and blocks. Some exhibit a high frequency of stuttering, while others exhibit very little overt stuttering possibly because they try to hide their speech disruptions. Some children stutter freely and openly and do not appear to be bothered by their disfluencies, while others stutter very little but are concerned about their speech. Put simply, there are just as many different ways to stutter as there are children who stutter.

In addition to these differences *between* children who stutter, there is also remarkable variability in stuttering *within* individual children who stutter. This variability can be seen from week to week, from day to day, and even from situation to situation (Yaruss 1997a), and the causes for this variability are numerous and not well understood. Throughout this book, we will explore some of the reasons that stuttering is so variable. For now, it is important to keep in mind that "what you see (or hear) is not always what you get" when observing school-age children who stutter.

One consequence of the variability between and within speakers is the fact that it may not be possible for you (or a pediatrician or a parent) to determine whether a child is stuttering by "taking a quick look" at a child's speech. Sometimes, of course, it is quite clear that a child stutters—you can see it in the speech disruptions, the tension, the struggle, or the negative impact these speech events have on the child's ability to interact with others or to succeed in school. Many times, however, it is harder to observe the stuttering behaviors because the child is hiding his stuttering or because he is stuttering less in that particular situation or on that particular day. To complicate matters further, a child who exhibits disruptions in speech may or may not need therapy—or be ready for it—at the time you conduct the initial evaluation. We simply cannot make that determination based solely on the behaviors the child exhibits during a brief observation. Determining whether a child actually stutters or needs therapy for stuttering requires that you have a solid understanding of what stuttering is and what it means to say that the child is a child who stutters.

What is stuttering?

In the history of the field of speech-language pathology, there have been literally dozens of definitions of stuttering posed by experts from both inside and outside of the field (Bloodstein 1993). One reason for all these different explanations is the variability of the disorder. When different authorities have looked at stuttering, they have looked at it from different perspectives based upon their own biases about communication, speech production, and human behavior. Thus, some theories about the nature of stuttering focus primarily on describing the physical behaviors involved in the moment of stuttering itself, while others focus more on the psychological or cognitive consequences of the speech disruptions. Still other theories have speculated about the possible cause(s) of the speech disruptions, such as differences in brain structure or function, various learning processes, or language-based difficulties.

Unfortunately, even with all this theorizing, we do not have a single, universally-agreed-upon definition of stuttering. Because of the vast differences of opinion about the nature of the disorder, it is possible that we may never have one. We also do not have a clear explanation for what causes stuttering, and again, this may prove elusive. Later in this chapter, we will provide an overview of our current understanding of the nature and causes of the disorder. But first, we will provide a "working definition" of stuttering that can guide us in answering the question of whether or not a child is stuttering. This working definition will help us view stuttering from a broad perspective, taking into account not only the observable characteristics of the child's speech, but also the many aspects of stuttering that may be hidden or "under the surface," such as the emotional and cognitive consequences of growing up with a speaking difficulty.

Stuttering is more than just stuttering.

One reason the term *stuttering* can be so confusing is the fact that it can be used to describe both a speech behavior and the speech disorder commonly associated with that behavior. In other words, we can use the term *stuttering* to refer to certain types of speech disruptions (e.g., repetitions, prolongations, blocks) and, at the same time, we can use the term *stuttering* to refer to the broader communication disorder. This communication disorder involves much more than just the observable speech disruptions; it also involves the *consequences* of the speech disruptions that the speaker may experience at multiple levels (e.g., tension and struggle, avoidance, emotional and cognitive reactions). Because the same term is used, it can be hard to know whether a given definition or theory is referring to the specific speech behaviors or to the broader communication disorder.

One helpful way of clarifying the different uses of the term *stuttering* is to maintain a clear distinction between *stuttering events* and the *stuttering disorder*. This is the strategy we will use throughout this book (i.e., We will use two working definitions of the term *stuttering*). Stuttering events are the speech disfluencies exhibited by many people who stutter. These disfluencies include repetitions, prolongations, and other interruptions in the forward flow of speech. (We will say more about the different types of disfluencies children produce in the next section, pages 13–14.) The stuttering *disorder*, on the other hand, refers to the entire experience the speaker may have due to the stuttering events. Thus, the stuttering disorder includes all of the feelings and emotions the child may experience because of stuttering, as well as any limitations the child may have in his ability to perform everyday speaking tasks and the disadvantages he may ultimately experience in his ability to achieve life goals (Yaruss 1998a).

Using these definitions, then, we can say the following about school-age children who stutter: Most children who stutter exhibit stuttering events. (We say *most* because there are some children who are so adept at hiding their stuttering that clinicians rarely hear any stuttering events in their speech.) A child might accomplish this by avoiding talking or by choosing his words carefully so he only tries to say those words he thinks he can say fluently. Similarly, most children who stutter also experience the stuttering disorder. Again, we say *most* because there are some children who stutter who experience relatively few negative consequences from their stuttering, even though they may exhibit stuttering events. (Indeed, this latter situation is the goal of speech therapy for many school-age children who stutter.) When working with children who stutter, therefore, we must consider both the observable stuttering events and the broader consequences that make up the stuttering disorder.

What are stuttering events?

Even this question is not easy to answer. Traditionally, stuttering events have been defined as those types of speech disfluencies that are typically produced by people who stutter (Conture 2001). This definition is not entirely satisfactory, however, for a number of reasons. First, research has demonstrated that it is difficult for the authorities in the field to reach agreement about which behaviors or events in a child's speech should be called stuttering (Cordes & Ingham 1995). Thus, a variety of different categorization schemes have been proposed in an attempt to differentiate stuttering from so-called "normal" disfluency (Yaruss 1997b). Although there are similarities between these classification systems, there are also some notable differences that can make it confusing for clinicians (and for families) to understand why some speech events may be called stuttering, while others may not. Second, there is no clear-cut distinction between the types of disfluencies exhibited by children who stutter and the types of disfluencies exhibited by children who do not stutter (Johnson & Associates 1959). In Chapter 3 on diagnostic strategies (pages 58–61), we will review in detail the specific types of disfluencies that are typically seen in the speech of children who stutter.

For now, it is important to recognize that all children produce all types of speech disfluencies, both those that are typically considered to be "normal" and those that are typically considered to be "stuttered" (Ambrose & Yairi 1999). Thus, all children exhibit the so-called "normal" disfluencies:

- phrase repetitions ("I want—I want that")

- revisions ("I want—I need that")

- interjections ("um," "er")

And all children exhibit the so-called "stuttered" (or "stutter-like" [Yairi 1996]) types of disfluencies:

- repetitions of sounds ("li-li-like this")

- prolongations ("llllike this")

- blocks ("l—ike this")

Furthermore, even those types of disfluencies that are typically considered "normal" can also be part of stuttering if a child exhibits physical tension during the disfluencies or uses them as a way of postponing or avoiding stuttering. Therefore, *the observable characteristics of the speech behaviors themselves cannot always be used solely to determine whether a speech disruption should be classified as a stuttering event.*

That said, it is true that we tend to see more of the so-called "stuttered" types of disfluencies in the speech of children who stutter (Ambrose & Yairi 1999; Yaruss, LaSalle, et al. 1998). Using the definitions presented above, we can say that "stuttering events are those types of disfluencies generally (though not exclusively) produced by people who stutter, and that these disfluencies tend to include repetitions of sounds or syllables, prolongations, and blocks."

What does it mean to say that a child stutters?

Another area that may cause confusion is whether a child who exhibits stuttering events in his speech should be labeled as a "child who stutters." In other words, how many "stutters" does it take to make a "stutterer?" Like many topics in the field of stuttering, this is a question that has caused a considerable amount of debate. Some clinicians apparently believe that any child who exhibits any stuttering events in his speech should be considered a child who stutters, while others apparently prefer to establish a minimum number of stuttering events that should be observed before the label of *stutterer* is applied. Still others determine whether a child should be considered a child who stutters based on factors other than the observable characteristics of stuttering.

So, as with so many questions in stuttering, there is no easy answer to this question of when to apply the label *child who stutters* to children exhibiting stuttering events. The situation is further complicated by concerns about the use of labels to identify children with communication difficulties, and also by individual preferences about the use of terms like *stutterer* and *child who stutters*. (See box below.) Our approach to this issue is again to maintain the distinction between stuttering events and the stuttering disorder using the working definitions presented previously. If a child exhibits stuttering events in his speech, then it seems reasonable to say that the child stutters—or is stuttering at that time. Whether or not that same child exhibits a stuttering disorder is

Is it "stutterer" or "child who stutters"?

Many of us have wondered whether we should refer to our students as *stutterers* or *children who stutter*. In fact, clinicians from many professions have struggled with the appropriate use of "person-first" language as a way of highlighting the value of the person, rather than focusing on the person's impairment or disability. The issue can evoke strong emotions on both sides, and clinicians may feel "caught in the middle," trying to use the right term.

Unfortunately, there is no simple answer. Although there has not been any research examining this issue in children, research with adults has shown that some speakers prefer to be called *people who stutter*—in part because it highlights the fact that stuttering is only a part of them—while others simply prefer *stutterer* (St. Louis 1999).

Because of these differences of opinion, we feel that it should be up to each individual, rather than society or the clinician, to determine which term is most comfortable. Given that some people seem to be very uncomfortable with the term *stutterer*, however, our rule of thumb is to use *person who stutters* or *child who stutters* in all situations, particularly if you do not know how the individual you are speaking with views the issue.

Regardless of the term that is used, we have found that, at an appropriate point in therapy, it is helpful to talk with the child about the terms that are used to refer to stuttering and to people who stutter. This is particularly important for older students, because it is an issue they will face throughout their lives. By helping our students become comfortable with these terms and discover their own preferences, we can help them develop coping skills they will need throughout their lives.

a different question, as is whether he sees himself as a person who stutters. To answer those questions, you will need to know much more about the child's feelings about his speech and the impact the stuttering events have on his ability to communicate and participate in life. Furthermore, the older a child gets, the more important it is to allow him to have a say in determining whether he should be considered a *child who stutters* or, indeed, whether he exhibits a stuttering "disorder" at all.

Myth: I'm not supposed to call it "stuttering."

Just as there are some people who stutter who are uncomfortable with the term *stutterer*, there are also those who are uncomfortable with the term *stuttering*. In this case, however, it seems to be clinicians who are uncomfortable using "the S-word" with their students.

It is likely that at least some of this discomfort traces back to older theories of stuttering that suggested, directly or indirectly, that people should not "draw attention" to a child's speaking difficulties (Johnson 1949). Thus, some clinicians and parents may prefer to use euphemisms such as "nonfluency" to describe disruptions in a child's speech. Still others may be uncomfortable "labeling" a child as stuttering if the speech disruptions may eventually resolve into normal speech (dis)fluency. (This is more often the case for preschool children.)

We agree that clinicians do not want to draw negative or unwanted attention to a child's speaking difficulties. As with all questions about the use of specific terminology to refer to people with communication disorders, it is important to keep in mind that it is not the word that matters so much as the intent with which the word is used. Also, as with all aspects of stuttering, there will be differences between individuals in how they prefer to refer to their speech.

If a child, family member, or teacher calls it *stuttering*, we do not encourage them to pick a different word. Rather than avoiding the word *stuttering*, we prefer to be straightforward with children about the name of their communication difficulty. We work to help them understand that *stuttering* is simply a term that is used to describe the interruptions in their speech. The more comfortable they can become with the term, the less likely they will be to react negatively when other people, such as teachers or peers, talk about their speech.

Therefore, we like to be flexible about the terms we use to describe stuttering. Generally, we ask the child what word he has used in the past to describe his speech and what words he would like to use now. Then we can use those words in therapy.

Doesn't everybody stutter sometimes?

Many times family members, teachers, and even clinicians will tell children that "everybody stutters sometimes" in an attempt to help them feel better about their speech. While we agree that we want children to feel comfortable with their speech, we do not think it is helpful to tell stuttering children that everybody stutters. This is especially true for older children and teens who can see that other people do not experience the same degree of tension, struggle, and discomfort that they experience when they try to speak. We do, however, want children to recognize that all people are disfluent. In fact, some apparently "normal" speakers exhibit a very high frequency of speech disfluencies. By making clear distinctions between speech disfluencies and stuttering events, and between stuttering events and the stuttering disorder, we can help children increase their understanding of their speaking difficulties and help them separate their stuttering from their reactions to their stuttering.

Why does *this* child stutter?

Throughout the history of our field, many different theories have been proposed about the cause of stuttering, and experts still disagree about which theory is best (Bloodstein 1993). Historically, theories have tended to focus on the idea that stuttering was "caused" by a specific factor such as a neurological tic, a psychological adjustment problem, deficits in linguistic ability or motor control, or environmental pressures or demands placed on the child. None of these theories has proven to be satisfactory, however, for they fail to adequately explain the observable symptoms of stuttering and the speaker's overall experience of the disorder. In essence, almost all of the historical theories tend to provide unidimensional explanations for what is clearly a multidimensional problem (Conture 2001).

Current theories take a different approach by stating that stuttering does not arise due to any single factor by itself. Instead, it has been proposed that stuttering results from an interaction among a number of different aspects of a child's development (Conture 2001, Smith & Kelly 1997, Starkweather & Givens-Ackerman 1997). Thus, rather than suggesting that stuttering is purely a motoric problem or a linguistic problem or a psychological problem, current theories suggest that stuttering is due to a complex interaction between these and other factors. These so-called "multifactorial" theories have significant promise for improving our understanding of the disorder, for they allow different factors to come into play for different children. This way of thinking helps us understand not only the variability of stuttering but also the fact that different children stutter in so many different ways.

It may not be possible for researchers to identify all of the factors associated with the development of stuttering; however, three of the factors most commonly implicated in current theories include:

- the child's language development
- the child's motoric abilities
- the child's personality or temperament

Note that each of these factors is partially determined by the child's environment and partially determined by the child's genes. This may explain the fact that stuttering tends to "run in families" but is not solely determined by genetic inheritance (Ambrose et al. 1993).

Note also that current theories do not suggest that children will stutter if they exhibit a deficit in one or more of the areas listed above. Rather, it is the *interaction* among factors that makes a child more or less prone to stutter. This underlying predisposition to stutter also interacts with the way the child attempts to use his language and motor skills when he is speaking. Because the child's speaking patterns are influenced by his environment, then the child's communication environment also plays an important role in the child's development of stuttering. Thus, in answer to the questions "Why is a child stuttering?" or "What causes stuttering?," we tell children and parents that *there are several factors involved, including factors inherent to the child and factors involving the child's environment*, and that *these factors interact in a complicated way* to make it more or less likely that a child will stutter.

Why doesn't he stutter all the time?

Stuttering is a highly variable and cyclic disorder. Children will stutter more on some days than on others, and more in some situations than in others. Sometimes, a child can tell when he's going to have a good day, and other times he may be taken by surprise, either by a period of relatively easy fluency or by a period of physically tense stuttering. We do not fully understand the causes of this variability, but we do know that the unpredictability of the disorder can make it very difficult for children to come to terms with their stuttering.

Myth: Stuttering is caused by . . .

When we are talking about stuttering with parents, teachers, family members, acquaintances, and even our young students themselves, we hear many different suggestions about what the cause of stuttering might be. Generally, these suggestions are presented as fact, even though they are based on an incomplete understanding of the disorder.

For example, we have been told that stuttering is caused by nervousness, excitement, parents being too hard on their children, children trying to "get attention," doing something wrong, something that happened when (or before) the child was born, brain damage, etc. Parents may even be concerned that their child might "catch" stuttering from another child who stutters, or they might have read that the stuttering was their fault because of how they raised their children.

The fact remains that the exact causes of stuttering are not entirely understood. Although a variety of theories have been proposed, there is still no "easy" answer to give the parents when they ask, "What caused this to happen?" *We do know that stuttering is not caused by nervousness, parents' behavior, brain damage, or any specific event that "happened" to the child.* These are myths that are often discussed in the general society, and propagating these myths does nothing to help children who stutter. As SLPs, we must take the lead and become advocates for changing these unfortunate misconceptions. In this way, we can help people who stutter by helping society understand the complexity of the disorder.

We can also help the children we work with—and the people in the children's environment—to develop a better understanding of what does *not* cause stuttering. Although they may initially be seeking a simple explanation for their problems, school-age children and others will be better able to handle the long-term consequences of the stuttering disorder when they understand that the causes of stuttering are complex and that stuttering is not anyone's fault.

Some days are "good" days. What are the other days?

As hard as it can be for the child who stutters to understand and accept the variability of the disorder, it may be even harder for other people in the child's life to accept. Parents are often confused when they see the stuttering "come and go." When they see the child being more fluent, they may express their hope that the child has finally "outgrown" the stuttering, only to be even more disappointed when the stuttering returns. They may think that the child is being lazy or trying to get attention during the more disfluent times, and they may wonder why the child doesn't just do more of whatever it was he was doing when he was fluent.

We believe that it is important for everyone, including the child, to accept the fact that variability is a normal part of the disorder. Throughout the child's entire life, he will experience variability in his speech. It is not necessary, or even particularly helpful, for the child or his parents to expend a lot of energy trying to figure out why the child is experiencing more or less stuttering in any given period of time. The more readily they can accept this variability as just a normal part of the stuttering disorder, the easier it will be for them to accept the stuttering itself.

Why does the child stutter more at home?

Often, children will seem to stutter more in certain situations than in others. Because of the variability mentioned above, we receive many questions from parents, children, teachers, and others about why a child stutters more in one place than another. As we have stated, there are no easy answers to these questions, though we do want to try to help everyone in the child's life understand the variability of stuttering.

A particularly common example of why it is essential that parents understand the variability of stuttering is seen in the case of the child who seems to stutter more at home. Parents and others can be confused about why this happens, and they may blame themselves for making the child uncomfortable or putting too much pressure on him. This added anxiety on the parents' part may actually cause them to put even more pressure on the child. To interrupt this cycle, we want to help parents understand that *they are not the cause of stuttering* and that *it is normal for the child's stuttering to vary*.

In many cases, we may also want to help the family realize that it can even be a good thing when a child stutters more at home than in other situations. This may indicate that the parents have created an atmosphere of acceptance where the child can feel comfortable with his speech and simply "be himself." Many times, a child may be tired of managing his stuttering all day while he is at school, so he may appreciate having a place where he is not expected to change the way he is speaking. It is also possible that the child is simply talking more (or more freely) at home than in other situations, and, as a result, is stuttering more.

We try to help people understand that there are a number of reasons why these "up and down" patterns of stuttering can develop. We may never really know why a child is experiencing more or less stuttering in a given situation or at a specific point in time. Regardless of whether we understand the reasons for the variability, however, the bottom line is simply that stuttering is a variable disorder.

Stuttering Is Variable

"The teacher sees it, but I don't."

John, age 8, was a second grader in a class of 22 students. His teacher, Mrs. M., approached me in the hall one day and asked me to "check" him when I had the chance. Later that day, I spoke with Mrs. M. during lunch and asked her to give me more information about the situation. She said she had observed John repeating words and sounds "a lot" when he started talking. I observed him the following day during a classroom discussion and a small group interaction. I did not observe any outward signs of stuttering. I told Mrs. M. that I would put him on my "check-back" list. Two days later, I came back to the classroom during a small group interaction. As I approached John's group, I noticed that he wasn't contributing much to the discussion. I began to ask him and the other children in the group a series of questions about their project. John stuttered moderately during this interaction.

The fact that I observed him in a variety of speaking situations gave me the information I needed to be able to observe his stuttering directly, refer him for evaluation, and eventually, recommend therapy.

Stuttering Is Variable

"I see it, but the teacher doesn't."

Callie, age 10, was a shy and quiet third grader. She had just transferred from another school into my district. About three weeks after her transfer, her mother called to let me know that Callie had a history of stuttering and that she had been dismissed from therapy at her last school because "her stuttering was mild and it didn't affect her academically."

Callie's mother reported that the transition to the new area and the new school had been difficult for Callie and that her stuttering "seemed to be getting worse."

After sending home the referral and paperwork, I sent a teacher checklist (see page 108) to her classroom teacher, Mr. G., to learn what he had been observing in the classroom. To my surprise, Mr. G. reported that Callie was doing "well" in the classroom and that he "had never heard her stutter."

Following up with an observation and a consult with the teacher, I asked the question, "How often does Callie raise her hand or talk in the classroom?" Mr. G. thought for a moment, and then replied, "You know, I never hear her talk very much. Maybe a word or two here or there."

During my assessment of Callie, I discovered that she had already become a master of hiding her stuttering and avoiding speaking situations. While it was also true that she had a shy disposition, her quietness had become part of her stuttering problem.

Even though Callie was a good student, her stuttering was holding her back socially and academically. In her academic settings, it was also keeping her from participating in classroom discussions. Because of the impact on her academic and social participation, she was clearly eligible for services under the Individuals with Disabilities Education Act (IDEA) 1997.

Callie is now in therapy and is realizing that stuttering is not as "bad" as she had thought, and that it is not something she needs to hide. Even though she is learning to manage her speech, she lets her stuttering out with less fear and embarrassment. She is talking more and is getting more out of her social and classroom interactions. Finally, she has become an advocate for "saying what she wants, when she wants, and to whom she wants."

Callie's teacher has also become quite adept at recognizing her avoidance tactics and works closely with me. He has been our best ally in the therapy process.

He's hiding his stuttering!

Some children who stutter are quite adept at hiding their stuttering behaviors. They can do this by changing the words they want to say when they feel they might stutter (circumlocution or "talking around" their point), or not participating in classroom discussions for fear of stuttering in front of their peers (avoidance).

People in the child's environments need to become aware of these avoidance behaviors and understand why the child is using them. Stuttering can be embarrassing, and if a child does not accept his stuttering, he may be more likely to try to hide it. Unfortunately, these avoidance tactics often have a much more disruptive effect on the child's communication than the stuttering itself.

Avoidance Behaviors

Mild stuttering can hold a child back.

Andrew, age 8, enjoys dinosaurs and building model kites. He was diagnosed with a "borderline to mild" stuttering disorder. In speech therapy, he was learning about his speech mechanism and about stuttering. His teacher became concerned that Andrew had begun to withdraw from social interactions and had stopped volunteering for any type of classroom speaking. During further probes about Andrew's communication attitudes, it was discovered that, despite Andrew's low frequency and severity of stuttering, he had developed extensive negative reactions to any disruptions in his speech. In therapy, we began to address these negative feelings while concurrently using desensitization strategies to help Andrew react less negatively to moments of stuttering.

Severe stuttering doesn't have to stop her.

Alicia, age 10, is a precocious girl who enjoys math competitions and talking on the phone to her friends. Her stuttering behaviors were labeled as "moderate to severe." In the classroom, Alicia volunteered to answer questions and was active in the drama and chorus. Alicia consistently struggled with her speech and exhibited a relatively high frequency of stuttering. Still, reflective writing and drawing activities revealed positive attitudes toward communication and self. Alicia's teacher was initially hesitant to call on her because "she took so long to answer," but through his collaboration with the SLP, the teacher learned strategies to help him be more patient and accepting of Alicia's stuttering. Her teacher learned to value Alicia's contributions in the classroom for what she was saying, rather than how she was saying it, and her increased classroom successes became a key component of her overall communication success. Because of these experiences, and because of Alicia's willingness to keep talking even though she stuttered, her teacher no longer hesitated to call on Alicia and Alicia improved her ability to manage her stuttering disorder.

In terms of avoidance behaviors, the connection between accurate assessment and effective therapy is apparent. When we look at his stuttering, we recognize that he is experiencing anxiety about his speech or having difficulty accepting his stuttering. As we will discuss later in the chapter on treatment strategies (Chapter 4), it will be important to address these fears in treatment by desensitizing the child to stuttering and helping him learn to accept his speech.

There are many ways children who stutter try to hide their stuttering. Here are some examples of the tricks our students have used:

- Talk r-e-al s-l-o-w
- I say "Never mind"
- don't answer the question
- Stop talking in class
- Hang up
- change a word
- Have parents or friends make phone calls
- Stay home from school when I have to give an oral report
- "Lose" my book when it's my turn to read

What you see is not always what you get.

Sometimes, teachers tell us that a child we are assessing or working with in therapy "doesn't stutter very much in the classroom." Our first question is always, "How much does the child talk in the classroom?" Just because we don't see the stuttering doesn't mean it's not happening, as the child may be hiding his stuttering.

In Chapter 3 (page 108–110), we present a teacher checklist we have used to gain information about a child's stuttering experiences in a classroom. It includes guiding questions that help a teacher make observations about avoidance behaviors and any other strategies a child may use to hide stuttering in the classroom. Gathering and discussing this information not only helps the teacher better understand the complexities of the stuttering disorder and the nature of the child's difficulties in communication, it also helps us better understand the issues we may need to address in treatment.

If a child is adept at hiding his stuttering in various situations, then it is likely that common measures, such as "stuttered syllables per minute" or the frequency of stuttering, will not provide a representative assessment of his stuttering behaviors in those situations (Cooper 1986). Therefore, when examining school-age children who stutter, we must ask ourselves whether stuttering counts can be truly representative with a child who uses hiding behaviors? In Chapter 3, we will discuss strategies for assessing the impact of the stuttering disorder on a child's communication by taking into account more than just stuttering counts.

Why is he *still* stuttering?

SLPs are familiar with the fact that many young children exhibit early signs of stuttering but do not go on to develop a lifelong stuttering problem. Research has demonstrated that many *preschool* children who exhibit early stuttering do ultimately develop into fluent speakers. In fact, as many as 75% of preschool children who stutter may develop fluent speech without intervention (Yairi & Ambrose 1999). (Note: It is not clear whether this high "recovery" rate applies to the population of preschool children who have stuttered for long enough that they were referred to an SLP for an evaluation or to the population of preschool children who stutter as a whole. At the very least, it most certainly does not apply to the population of school-age children being discussed in this book.)

Not all stuttering preschoolers "grow out of it," however. At least 25% of preschool children who stutter (and perhaps a higher percentage of those evaluated by SLPs) will continue to stutter as school-age children, adolescents, and even adults. Ultimately, those preschool children who do not "grow through" their stuttering at an early age (before approximately age 7) are at an increased risk for developing chronic stuttering.

Remember that the notion that many preschoolers develop out of a period of stuttering does not apply to the school-age population we are addressing in this book. Furthermore, we cannot predict, with absolute certainty, which preschool children will develop out of their early stuttering and which preschoolers will become school-age children who stutter (Conture 2001). Therefore, we believe that *appropriate early intervention is critical for preschool children who stutter.* Although there is considerable disagreement among experts about how long to wait before recommending treatment (Curlee & Yairi 1997, Zebrowski 1997, Bernstein Ratner 1997), *we prefer to enroll preschool children in an appropriate form of intervention sooner rather than later.*

Why didn't this child outgrow it?

Given the current level of knowledge in the field, we cannot definitively answer the question of why some children continue to stutter past the preschool years. We do have some research that provides certain "red flags" or warning signs indicating that a preschool child is at increased risk for continuing to stutter. Generally, when we are working with a school-age child who stutters, one or more of the risk factors shown in the box on the next page have been present.

Keep in mind that this list, which has been drawn from several sources, indicates "at-risk" factors, not "causal" factors. In other words, we cannot look at any one or two of these factors and say, without question, that they are the reason a particular child continued to stutter. Instead, these are examples of the types of factors we consider when we are making a decision about whether a preschool child is likely to need treatment based on whether he is likely to continue stuttering. It also may help gain a better understanding of the child's experience of stuttering.

Some Risk Factors that May Indicate that Preschool Children Who Stutter Should Be Enrolled in Therapy

1. **There is a history of persistent stuttering in the family.** There is a genetic component to stuttering, so stuttering tends to run in families. Preschool children who have relatives who stutter are at a greater risk for continuing to stutter (Ambrose et al. 1993).

2. **The child exhibits more "stuttered" disfluencies than "normal" disfluencies.** Because all children exhibit all types of disfluencies, it can be difficult to tell whether a preschool child who exhibits speech disfluencies is actually at risk for stuttering. The proportion of stuttered versus normal disfluencies can sometimes provide an indication about the child's risk level (Conture 2001).

3. **The child has been stuttering for six months or more.** Most preschool children who are ultimately going to recover from early stuttering do so within the first six months, though some young children do recover from early suttering within the first year or even two years since the onset of stuttering (Yairi & Ambrose 1999).

4. **The child is aware of or concerned about his speech disfluencies.** Awareness of stuttering may cause a child to become self-conscious about his speaking difficulties. As a result, he may try various strategies to "fix" his stuttering (e.g., using increased physical tension or struggle) that actually result in an increase in the severity of his stuttering (Logan & Yaruss 1999).

5. **The child has developed fears or avoidance reactions to stuttering.** Avoidance behaviors, such as changing words (circumlocution), not talking in certain situations, and other internal reactions, can cause children to "shut down" or "withdraw" from social situations (Manning 2001).

6. **Parents and others have reacted negatively to the child's stuttering.** Although parental behavior definitely does not cause stuttering, the reactions of the people in a child's environment can affect the child's perceptions about speaking and stuttering (Bernstein Ratner 1993).

7. **The child has concomitant speech or language deficits.** Children with other communication disorders *in addition to stuttering* appear to be at greater risk for continuing to stutter. Therefore, they may be more likely to require therapy (Yairi et al. 1996).

27

Wait and see?

By the time a child reaches the school-age years (older than approximately age 7), he is highly unlikely to spontaneously develop "normal" fluency (Andrews & Harris 1964). The reasons for this are not entirely clear. The chronic nature of stuttering for most school-age children may be associated with the genetic nature of the disorder, or it may simply be due to the fact that the speaking and stuttering patterns become ingrained in children's speech. An 8-year-old child who began to experience disruptions at age three and a half has spent well more than half his life stuttering, so it is not entirely surprising that the stuttering is just part of the way he speaks. Regardless of the reason the stuttering stays, however, the bottom line is that "wait and see" is no longer sound advice for school-age children who stutter.

Do I Need to Refer Him to Somebody Else?

Occasionally, we hear specialists or others say that SLPs (particularly school-based SLPs) are not the right professionals to treat stuttering. Put simply, we disagree. Children who stutter are best served by qualified clinicians who care about the development of effective communication. SLPs are the professionals who understand the most about the stuttering disorder and about helping children develop effective communication skills. Plus, we believe that children who stutter need us!

What about other disciplines?

Sometimes, stuttering may look like a disorder of nervousness, anxiety, or some other psychological issue. In fact, some clinicians and parents may wonder whether a referral to a psychologist or counselor is necessary when treating school-age children who stutter. It is certainly true that outside referrals are necessary if a child exhibits mental health issues aside from stuttering, if the child's concerns about stuttering are too severe, or if you do not feel capable of appropriately working with the child's emotions. Furthermore, counselors, physicians, and others can be helpful colleagues for collaboration on a case-by-case basis. For the majority of cases, however, SLPs are the professionals who are most qualified to deal with the emotional issues and other concerns related to stuttering, for we are the professionals who know and understand stuttering events, the stuttering disorder, and people who stutter.

28

Where do I go for help?

Throughout this book, we will refer to various resources that provide additional information about stuttering and stuttering treatment. A summary of these resources can also be found in Appendix 2A, pages 45 and 46. It is our belief that familiarizing ourselves with these resources is an integral part of the process of developing advanced clinical skills and increasing our confidence levels in our abilities to help children who stutter.

Many of the available resources are targeted specifically at providing education and emotional support for children who stutter and their families. These resources support our clinical services by providing helpful materials we can give to families who are seeking additional information about their children's speech. In addition, there are also many resources focused on helping SLPs. Organizations such as the Stuttering Foundation of America (SFA) and the National Stuttering Association (NSA) have developed numerous publications and continuing education programs that are devoted to helping SLPs improve their clinical skills and confidence levels in the diagnosis and treatment of stuttering. In addition, there are many expert clinicians in our profession who have dedicated their careers to increasing clinicians' understanding of stuttering and stuttering therapy. These colleagues and resources are available and we should not hesitate to take advantage of them. We do not have to be alone.

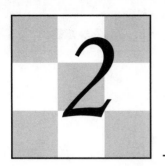

How Do I Begin?

Preparing Ourselves for Success

Once you have made the decision to work on developing your skills for working with children who stutter, the next task is to evaluate your current understanding of stuttering and consider some new ways of looking at the disorder. In this chapter, we will explore some common preconceptions clinicians have about stuttering and provide some new perspectives to help SLPs feel more confident about their skills in this area.

I remember something about stuttering from school, but . . .

We believe that it is important for clinicians to have a thorough understanding of the stuttering disorder. Still, many clinicians tell us that their courses in stuttering were mostly about theory and that they are not certain where to start in the clinic. They say that they remember hearing that stuttering is confusing and that it's harder to treat than other disorders, but they don't remember learning many specific goals or strategies they can use in therapy. While the complexity of stuttering can make therapy challenging at times, it is important to remember that *it is possible – and probable – for successful and effective stuttering therapy to occur in many settings.*

By and large, the textbooks of today are very different from those of the past, and many contain a wealth of practical situations about how to help people who stutter. It is a good idea to have at least one recently published text in your collection of reference materials. These new resources allow you to combine theory with practice and ensure that your treatment is based on sound theoretical principles. Several recent texts and other valuable resources are listed in Appendix 2A, pages 45 and 46.

Is stuttering really *that* different from other disorders?

Many experts have emphasized the notion that stuttering is a challenging disorder to treat. While this is true, we believe that clinicians *can* become comfortable with treating stuttering, and that they can do this by drawing on many of the skills they already possess. Indeed, we approach many of the speech management aspects of stuttering therapy in much the same way we approach articulation and language therapy. As SLPs, we already know how to manipulate factors such as linguistic complexity and environmental demands to help children achieve success with new target skills. As noted above, we often start new concepts at the word level, and then move to the phrase level, sentence level, and, finally, multi-sentence levels. Ultimately, we then move the child toward improved skills in conversational speech. The same process of using hierarchies to introduce new concepts applies to many aspects of stuttering therapy.

SLPs can also draw upon their considerable experience with language therapy, training with speech sound disorders, and working with children with autism. Regardless of the specific nature of a child's communication disorder, we know that we must make therapy meaningful for each child on our caseload. Likewise, examples and exercises in stuttering therapy must be based on experiences from the child's world, rather than on abstract concepts and procedural instructions. Also, as in all types of therapy, we know that we cannot wait for perfection in the therapy room before we move into "real world" settings if we wish to enhance carryover and generalization. Rather, we help children incorporate new skills into their daily lives from very early on in the treatment process. All of these concepts, which we already know from treatment with other disorders, are a part of successful stuttering therapy. This is true for many other techniques and strategies that are already second-nature to practicing SLPs.

Finally, working with the various other disorders we treat has helped us refine our skills for collaborating with parents and teachers to increase carryover and long-term success. These skills will be among the most crucial elements of treatment when we are working with children who stutter.

What we have been told about stuttering

There are many myths about stuttering. We are going to try to dispel some of these myths. Our aim is to provide you with specific knowledge to combat common myths, as well as sample language you can use to explain the basis for these myths to students and their families. We want to help you advocate for increased understanding about how these myths came into being and why they no longer stand up to scrutiny, given what we now know about stuttering.

First, we will discuss some of the ideas about stuttering therapy and about our ability to treat stuttering successfully that have been discussed within our own profession. We want to highlight just a few of the "old truths" and offer a set of newer, more positive realities.

1. **"There is no cure."** We often hear parents, teachers, and children who stutter lament the fact that there is no cure for stuttering. In fact, this is *one* "old truth" that is also a current reality. It is important for us to acknowledge this fact openly and honestly, even though it may be uncomfortable for some to hear. We know that we can help children with certain voice, articulation, and language problems completely overcome their speaking difficulties. For some reason that is still unknown, however, we cannot do this with the vast majority of school-age children who stutter. This fact can be hard for many clinicians to accept. It is also hard for parents, family members, and teachers to understand, for they may continue to hope that the child will simply outgrow the problem and suddenly begin to exhibit normal speech fluency.

   Unfortunately, there are still people in the world who will promise a cure for stuttering. For obvious reasons, many families are willing and eager to believe these promises. As SLPs with specific expertise in the area of stuttering, however, we must be the first line of defense to help families who may be shopping around for something that is not attainable. This is why we discuss with everyone who is involved with our students the fact that there is no cure for stuttering in school-age children. Of course, they also need to understand that the lack of a cure does *not* mean that a stuttering child will not improve. Indeed, families must learn that children who stutter *can* improve their speech, their ability to interact with others, and their overall communication skills. Through treatment and support, children who stutter can learn to improve all of these aspects of communication so stuttering will have a minimal impact on their lives.

2. **"Children who stutter never get better."** Sometimes, people in a child's environment mistakenly believe that the only acceptable form of improvement is the attainment of so-called "normal" fluency. Thus, once they learn that there is no cure for stuttering, they may mistakenly believe that children who stutter never get better. Unfortunately, we have heard such statements from many sources, including parents, teachers, clinicians, administrators, and even some children who stutter.

   It is true that in the absence of therapy, most school-age children who stutter do not simply "get better." With therapy, however, a child can make significant gains in her ability to speak more fluently and to communicate freely and easily. Of course, even with successful treatment, some stuttering is likely to remain in the child's speech. Thus, people who are expecting a complete recovery may feel that the child has not gotten any better.

   If we look at success in a unidimensional way, and if we believe that the only successful outcome of stuttering therapy is perfectly fluent speech, then we are creating an unrealistic expectation that will cause us to view our clients—and ourselves—as failures. As we change our own thinking about stuttering to a framework that allows us to view successes in new ways, we can work to change this perception in others in the child's environment, such as our colleagues, students, and families. Ultimately, the child and the those around her will recognize the many ways children who stutter CAN and DO get better as the result of effective stuttering therapy.

3. **"Easy starts and slow speech are the answer."** Easy onset of phonation ("easy starts") and a slower rate of communication are important tools for helping children improve their speech fluency. Nevertheless, this is not where we begin in therapy, and it is certainly not where we end. If we only teach the child how to manage speech and keep it "fluent," then we are helping the child deal with only a small piece of the puzzle. In addition to learning how to minimize tension in her muscles during speech, the child must also learn what to do with the tension she is already experiencing in her speech muscles. This is how she can learn to successfully manage both fluency and stuttering.

Although it is true that many children do speak more fluently when they speak more slowly, slowing speech rate does *not* need to be a direct goal of therapy. "Slowing down" is a relatively simplistic description of a multitude of factors involved in speaking. The relationship between speaking rate and speech fluency is highly complex. It is our bias that decreased rate of speech is a *by product* of many of the management tools that we discover with children in therapy. Therefore, as we discuss in more detail in Chapter 4, focusing on a broader set of management strategies gives the child a more comprehensive and flexible collection of tools than simply working on decreased speaking rate.

4. **"We cannot successfully treat stuttering in the schools."** Many school-based clinicians have heard and, in some cases, actually come to believe that they cannot effectively help children who stutter. Our field's track record from the "old days" contributes to this pessimistic belief as well as the negative thought processes that accompany it.

It is true that historically, many people who stuttered did not receive optimal therapy from their school-based clinicians. Today, however, the truth is that stuttering *can* be appropriately treated in the schools. Children who stutter *need* school clinicians! School-based clinicians may be the first speech professionals many children who stutter ever encounter. If we are not a part of the solution, we may become part of the problem.

Successful school-based stuttering therapy happens every day. Even if a clinician does not feel completely comfortable with her skills for helping children who stutter, she can still provide helpful services to her students. We have to remember that our students are on a journey to becoming effective communicators. We, too, are on that journey. We cannot expect perfection from our students and they, in turn, cannot expect it from us. As we grow in our skills and as well learn about the best ways to deal with stuttering for each individual student, we will become the most successful clinicians we can be.

5. **"We are not good enough to treat stuttering."** Unfortunately, another common message clinicians receive is that they do not have adequate skills for treating children who stutter. We feel

that the field of fluency disorders has done itself a significant disservice in propagating this myth. Of course, it couldn't be further from the truth—a clinician does not have to devote his or her entire career to stuttering in order to be a successful stuttering therapist.

Still, it may be true that we have not been trained well enough to treat stuttering successfully. This brings us to our biggest dilemma. As SLPs, we have often been told that we are supposed to know everything about everything in the communication realm. Unfortunately, nobody can accomplish this lofty goal. Due in part to the dramatically increasing scope of practice in communication science and disorders, stuttering is no longer emphasized in many university training programs. The number of programs offering in-depth training in fluency is decreasing even further. Because university training programs can only prepare us for so much during a two-year masters degree, a significant portion of the learning we need to do must happen "on the job."

For some of the disorder areas we treat regularly, we can gain this post-graduate education and experience relatively quickly. For areas such as stuttering, however, it may take some time before we feel competent and confident about our clinical skills. Feeling concerned about treating children who stutter does *not* mean that we "aren't good enough." It means that we need good continuing education and resources to help us improve our skills. In any case, no matter how good we are at anything, it is always the "best practice" to keep current and to gain insight from many different sources of information and viewpoints.

What we know about ourselves

SLPs are creative. It has been said that kindergarten teachers and SLPs are among the most creative professionals in the education arena. We can turn a stroll in the hallway into a therapy session and we can turn a broom closet into a therapy room. Our creativity can help us enhance the stuttering therapy experience we provide for our students and ourselves.

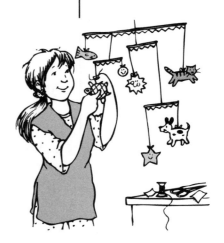

SLPs are clinical problem solvers. Whatever obstacles we face, we can overcome them using our clinical problem-solving skills. When we think about some of the challenges SLPs face on a day-to-day basis, we are constantly impressed by the variety of problem solving we see and creative solutions we find. Not enough time for therapy? We have seen SLPs flex their schedules and bring children in before the school day begins. Not certain what to do next? SLPs brainstorm about new directions with the child or call a colleague to get new ideas. The SLP's ability to solve these and other problems provides a positive example for the children they serve, for they are modeling problem-solving strategies that will help children become long-term "managers" of their own communication skills.

On page 31, we talked about the similarities between helping children who stutter and children with other speech and language disorders. You have a wealth of knowledge and skills that are already in place to help you become successful in treating stuttering. Therefore, when approaching stuttering therapy, keep in mind your existing skills for collaboration, fostering transfer and generalization, modeling target behaviors for children and parents, building hierarchies, and helping children build self-esteem.

SLPs know how to interact with children. Children are very special. We know this and we have a great foundation for relating with them. A child who stutters is no different from any other child on your caseload. She needs you to understand that *she* is not her *stuttering*, that she is a whole person, and that this "problem" is only a part of her life. When you use your interpersonal skills, you develop a rapport with a child that goes beyond any techniques or tools. Then, you can move away from being a speech technician to being a true *clinician* who understands the child's needs and, as a result, treats the child's stuttering more effectively.

SLPs know how to listen. It is true that SLPs are good talkers. (Just get a group of SLPs together and try to get in a word!) Importantly, we are also good listeners—or we are learning to become better listeners. We know that good communication is not just about talking; it is also about *listening* effectively. Children who stutter need a safe place to talk about their stuttering and how they feel about it with somebody who will *listen.* Our active listening skills will provide an environment where a child can feel comfortable talking about any topic related to her stuttering, not just about how much she is using her "speech tools."

SLPs are communication specialists. If we don't treat stuttering, who will? Stuttering is not a psychological disorder (regardless of what some classification systems may suggest), and it is not simply a disorder of movement. Stuttering is a disorder of *communication*, and we are the communication specialists. We understand the importance of being able to say "what you want, when you want, and to whom you want." Whether the message is fluent or not is not the only goal. Who else in a child's environment will ever give her THAT message?

Changing our thinking

The biggest obstacle that keeps many SLPs from achieving success in treating stuttering is a vicious cycle that we have created for ourselves. This cycle not only affects our thinking about our abilities to treat stuttering, it also keeps us from recognizing our strengths. This uncertainty about our abilities leads to decreased confidence, which leads to greater discomfort with stuttering treatment and, ultimately, with stuttering itself. We have spent some time in the past few pages trying to outline the compelling ways we can increase our comfort levels.

The figures on the next page show two trains of thought for an SLP. The first set of thoughts has an aspect of negativity that can prevent us from making progress in our own goals to become more effective in treating stuttering. The second set of thoughts represents a more positive spin on the challenges of stuttering therapy.

Appendix 2B on page 47 is an exercise adapted from the Stuttering Foundation of America's workbook entitled *The School-Age Child Who Stutters: Working Effectively with Attitudes and Emotions* (Chmela & Reardon 2001). We have adapted the task to demonstrate how we, as clinicians, can change our own thinking about our abilities to successfully treat stuttering. (See also Ramig & Bennett 1997).

Changing Our Thinking

Negative
Thinking

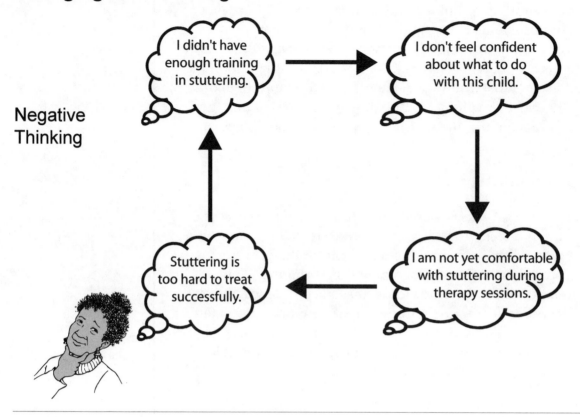

Positive
Thinking

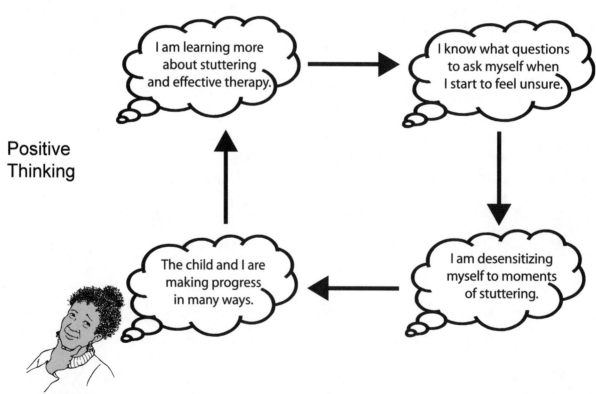

Schools Alert: I can't do all this; I work in the schools!

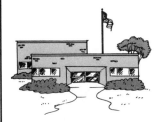

School-based SLPs are faced with many demands on their time and resources so they may feel particularly uncomfortable with stuttering. Still, the schools can be an ideal setting for helping children who stutter. So much of a child's daily communication happens at school, so working in the school allows greater opportunities for fostering carryover and generalization of speaking tools and positive communication attitudes. Often, peers and even siblings are readily available to be partners in therapy sessions. Furthermore, school-based clinicians have direct access to the child's teachers so they can draw upon information from the child's curriculum for materials to be used in therapy.

We have found that school-based therapy can be most successful when clinicians select treatment goals that are focused on the entire stuttering disorder, rather than just the observable stuttering events. While it can be difficult to establish new habits for using speech modification tools in the limited amount of time available for therapy in many schools, it is quite possible to use the available time to help children learn about and understand their stuttering and, ultimately, to come to accept their speech so they can become more effective communicators.

School-based SLPs are extremely dedicated and creative individuals who care about what is best for the children they serve. Clinicians can overcome any perceived obstacle to effective treatment if they remember that they are not alone in their frustrations, and that they are not alone in determining how to turn challenges into opportunities.

Private Sector Alert: I can't do all this; I work at a hospital/private practice!

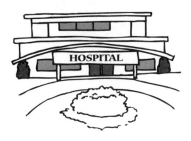

Even though the challenges may be different from those in the schools, private-sector SLPs also face a number of difficulties in the treatment of stuttering. Increasingly, clinicians face the pressures of third-party payment and reimbursement as a limiting factor in the duration and type of treatment they provide. Private-sector clinicians may also have limited access to many of the child's "real-world" situations, such as school and home. Thus, they need to work even harder to foster generalization of their client's speaking skills. Ultimately, however, even these obstacles can be overcome with creativity, collaboration with other professionals, and through partnership with parents and others to enhance the effectiveness of therapy that takes place in a setting that is not representative of a child's daily communication environment.

Preparing Our Children for Success

I worked with a child who stuttered a few years ago. Won't it just be the same treatment?
No two children who stutter are the same. This is a fact that we will repeat again and again throughout this book. One reason we place so much emphasis on the differences between children who stutter is that we want clinicians to recognize that treatment must be tailored to the needs of each individual child. We do not feel that clinicians can simply use the same set of treatment goals or the same set of treatment strategies for every student they see.

What is successful therapy?
The goal of speech therapy is for children who stutter to be able to communicate freely. Some authors have phrased this goal as children "being able to say what they want to say when they want to say it" (Conture & Guitar 1993). Although improved speech fluency is certainly a part of this equation, it is not the entire picture. Successful therapy is therapy that helps children communicate freely and participate in their daily lives. To achieve this, clinicians must do more than simply teach fluency techniques. They must also do more than simply teach children to accept their stuttering. Successful therapy involves a *balance* between fluency, stuttering, and attitudes.

Is it *really* okay to stutter?
Part of our role as clinicians is to help children who stutter gain more control over their speech, and, as a result, increase their level of fluency. Still, it is imperative that we do not allow ourselves (or our students) to view success or failure as being solely determined by the amount of fluent speech they produce. If we determine our progress based only on stuttering counts, we essentially ignore the fact that stuttering is highly variable over time and across situations. Even though a child may be able to achieve a low stuttering count in one situation, this does not necessarily mean that she will be able to do the same in another situation.

Furthermore, as noted previously, there is no cure for stuttering. So even after successful therapy, children may continue to exhibit some stuttering in their speech. If they are going to be able to accept themselves as speakers and as effective communicators, they must be able to tolerate that remaining stuttering. We have to help children (and ourselves) learn and understand that it really is okay to stutter.

Myth: We're "Speech" Therapists.
We're Supposed to Fix Their Speech!

Throughout this chapter, we have emphasized the notion that stuttering involves more than just speech disfluencies. This fact not only affects the child's experience of the stuttering disorder, it also affects our treatment of the disorder. If we accept the fact that most school-age children who stutter are unlikely to completely eliminate their productions of speech disfluencies (Andrews & Harris 1964), then we also need to accept the fact that *we* cannot be expected to fix the child's speech. We cannot teach children a simple trick that will magically make them become completely fluent all the time. Furthermore, although we can teach them strategies that will help them speak more fluently, we cannot ensure that children will use their fluency modification techniques at all times, in all situations. Thus, what we can do is help children learn how to be the best communicators they can possibly be, and we can give them the support and the tools they will need so they will not be held back by their stuttering. Though this is not a "fix" for their stuttering (in that they may still exhibit some stuttering events), it does result in a significant reduction in the frequency of their stuttering behaviors, the severity of their disfluencies, and most notably, in the negative consequences of the stuttering disorder. Therefore, stuttering may no longer cause a problem for them, even though they are still stuttering somewhat.

It can be difficult for us as clinicians to maintain our conviction about the broad nature of goals of stuttering therapy when so many of the people around us are expecting us to simply fix the child's speech. Parents, teachers, other SLPs, and even some authorities on stuttering appear to take the view that all children who stutter should be able to completely overcome their speaking difficulties and speak normally in all situations. Unfortunately, most research does not support this claim, and this view essentially places a lot of blame and burden on SLPs (and children who stutter) for not being able to cure an incurable condition.

For this reason, we supplement goals for improving children's speech fluency with goals for improving communication attitudes and interaction skills. We do not focus exclusively on fluency. Furthermore, we spend a lot of time educating others about stuttering and making certain that the people in our student's environment understand the broad-based nature of therapy and that the child's speech may still include some (milder) stuttering even after therapy is successfully completed.

Finally, so much of the stuttering disorder involves the cognitive and affective reactions to the stuttering events themselves. As Wendell Johnson (1961) once said, "Stuttering . . . is what the stutterer does trying not to stutter." In other words, much of the tension and struggle observed during stuttering can be traced from the speaker's (unsuccessful) attempts to control her speech. Therefore, if a child is trying to achieve "perfect fluency" (a condition that does not actually exist, since all speakers are disfluent to some extent), then the pressure of trying to achieve that unattainable goal can contribute to the child's negative affective and cognitive reactions to stuttering. This will result in more tension in the speaking mechanism, and ultimately, in more stuttering. Therefore, far from "giving up" on a child's fluency, accepting the fact that it is okay to stutter can actually help children reduce their stuttering and speak more fluently. The flowcharts on pages 48 and 49 (Appendix 2C) are useful to illustrate the thinking associated with how a child can accept the fact that she stutters.

What do you mean "affective and cognitive reactions?"
The beliefs and feelings children have about themselves as communicators can have a substantial impact on how well they are able to progress in therapy and how well they will learn to cope with stuttering throughout their lives (Manning 2001). *Dealing with these emotional components of stuttering is a central part of the therapy process.* Unfortunately, many clinicians tell us that they do not feel comfortable with their skills in this area. This is understandable, since most SLPs have not been formally trained about the emotional consequences of many communication disorders, including stuttering. In later chapters, we will discuss specific strategies for helping children understand and, ultimately, cope with their feelings and beliefs about stuttering. We will also review a number of resources you can consult to further develop your own skills for helping people who stutter address the emotional consequences of stuttering.

The "Good" Stutterer: Sending the Right Messages

We have discussed the fact that many clinicians have been taught that the goal of stuttering therapy is perfectly fluent speech. We have also discussed the problems that can be created when this is presented as the only acceptable outcome of therapy. By setting an unattainable goal, we are setting ourselves (and the child) up for failure and we are teaching our students that they should feel inadequate and unsuccessful every time they experience a moment of stuttering. Because most school-age children who stutter are likely to continue stuttering in some fashion throughout their lives, we need to be very careful about the messages we send regarding self-acceptance and about our own acceptance of children's stuttering.

When we praise children who stutter only for their fluent speech (as opposed to praising them also for successful communication), we are indirectly sending the message that their stuttered speech is not acceptable. If we do not allow children to explore their stuttering within the supportive environment of therapy, we may be inadvertently sending them the message that it is not okay to stutter in any setting. Though this may not be the message we intend to send, we must be aware that *what we say is not always what children hear.*

We want children who stutter to feel good about themselves and their communication skills, both when they are fluent and when they are stuttering. To do this, we must help ourselves, and those in the child's environment, to become aware of the fact that we can send positive or negative messages about the child's speech by what we say and what we do.

What messages am I sending?

As we work with children who stutter, we must consider the messages we may be sending about their speech. Here are some examples:

"Jason seems to be having a 'bad' speech day today." It is true that a child who stutters experiences variability in the amount of stuttering he experiences on a day-to-day basis. He also experiences variability in the amount of control he is able to achieve over his physical tension when speaking and in his ability to use tools to improve his fluency. These are natural variations that are associated with many different factors, most of which are beyond the child's control. When we judge a child's speech as "good" or "bad" based on such factors, we send the message that the only acceptable speech is fluent speech. Also, because the child may not know why he is experiencing greater or lesser fluency on a given day, we end up praising him (or criticizing him) for something he didn't actually intend to do. Thus, not only does this message have possible negative consequences for the child's self-esteem, it also does not make sense from a behavioral standpoint.

You can help parents learn how to reframe the messages they are sending to their children about stuttering by modeling appropriate responses. For example, when we hear parents say something like, "Kyle's speech is really bad today," we try to respond in a way that shows them a different way of talking about speech, such as, "So what I hear you saying is that Kyle is having more stuttering today." Or a parent might say, "Annie's speech is so much worse lately!" Our response is, "I can hear your concern. Please tell me about what you are seeing that makes you feel Annie's speech is getting worse."

Chapter 2

You can also reframe messages for the child if she says something like, "I don't want to do voluntary stuttering with strangers. I'm too nervous." Our response is, "I hear that you don't feel ready to do voluntary stuttering with people you don't know. I'm wondering what I can do to help you feel more comfortable." These types of responses and activities are discussed further in Chapter 4.

"Lucy, you did a 'great job' today!" A child who stutters needs to be validated and praised for her efforts in speech therapy. Still, we must be careful to offer our encouraging praise for all types of speech and for all types of progress in therapy. This includes gains in affective and cognitive components as well as improvements in willingness to communicate in difficult situations. In order for us to send a child the right message about her speech, we do not say that she did a "great job" only when she exhibits "less stuttering." We also highlight the fact that she did a great job when taking risks with communication, trying new management techniques (for speech fluency or for communication attitudes), self-advocating, and even for letting her stuttering "show" or for stuttering more openly.

Stuttering and Counseling Skills Resources

Organizations

American Speech-Language-Hearing
Association (ASHA)
10801 Rockville Pike
Rockville, MD 20852
1-800-638-8255
www.asha.org

Friends: The Association for Young People
Who Stutter
1220 Rosita Road
Pacifica, CA 94044
1-866-866-8335
www.friendswhostutter.org

National Stuttering Association (NSA)
4071 E. LaPalma Ave., Suite A
Anaheim, CA 92807
1-800-We-Stutter (800-937-8888)
www.WeStutter.org
e-mail: info@WeStutter.org

✓ *Our Voices: Inspirational Insights From
Young People Who Stutter* by A. Bradberry
and N. Reardon

✓ *Preschool Children Who Stutter: Information
and Support for Parents* (2nd Ed.) by J. S.
Yaruss and N. Reardon

Stuttering Foundation of America (SFA)
P.O. Box 11749
3100 Walnut Grove Road #603
Memphis, TN 38111
1-800-992-9392
www.stutteringhelp.org
e-mail: stutter@stutteringhelp.org

✓ *The School-Age Child Who Stutters: Working
Effectively With Attitudes and Emotions*
K. Chmela and N. Reardon

Websites

The Stuttering Home Page
www.stutteringhomepage.com

Information about Becoming a Board
Recognized Specialist in Fluency Disorders
www.ausp.memphis.edu/sbfd

Journal Articles

Counseling Parents of Children Who Stutter.
American Journal of Speech-Language Pathology.
P.M. Zebrowski and R. L. Schum 1993, 2, 65-
73.

Facing the Challenge of Treating Stuttering
in the Schools (Part I: Selecting Goals and
Strategies for Success). *Seminars in Speech and
Language.* J. Scott Yaruss (Ed.). 2002, 23(3)

Facing the Challenge of Treating Stuttering in
the Schools (Part II: One Size Does Not Fit
All). *Seminars in Speech and Language.*
J. Scott Yaruss (Ed.). 2003, 24(1)

Books

Applications of Counseling in Speech-Language Pathology and Audiology
T. Crowe

Ben Has Something to Say: A Story About Stuttering
L. Lears

Clinical Decision Making in Fluency Disorders (2nd Ed.)
W. Manning, Singular/Thompson Learning

Family-Based Treatment in Communicative Disorders: A Systematic Approach (2nd ed).
J. Andrews and M. Andrews, Janelle Publications, Inc.

How to Talk So Kids Will Listen and Listen So Kids Will Talk (20th Anniversary Edition)
A. Faber and E. Mazlish

The Nature and Treatment of Stuttering: New Directions (2nd ed.).
R. F. Curlee and G. M. Siegel (Eds.)

The Skilled Helper: A Problem-Management and Opportunity-Development Approach to Helping (7th Ed.)
G. Egan

Stuttering: An Integrated Approach to its Nature and Treatment (2nd ed.)
B. Guitar

Stuttering and Other Fluency Disorders
F. H. Silverman

Stuttering and Related Disorders of Fluency (2nd ed.)
R. F. Curlee (Ed.)

Stuttering: Its Nature, Diagnosis, and Treatment
E. G. Conture

Stuttering Therapy: Rationale and Procedures
H. H. Gregory, J. H. Campbell, C. B. Gregory, and D. G. Hill

Successful Stuttering Management Program (SSMP): For Adolescent and Adult Stutterers (2nd Ed)
D. H. Breitenfeldt and D. R. Lorenz

Synergistic Stuttering Therapy: A Holistic Approach
C.M. Bloom and D. K. Cooperman

Changing Our Thinking: An Activity for Clinicians

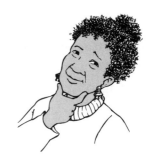

List some of the negative things you say to yourself about your ability to treat stuttering. Then reframe the thought and parallel each one with a more positive statement.

Negative	Positive

This illustration demonstrates the negative effects that can happen when Angela, age 10, is not accepting of her stuttering. When she tries to hide stuttering, she may end up stuttering more!

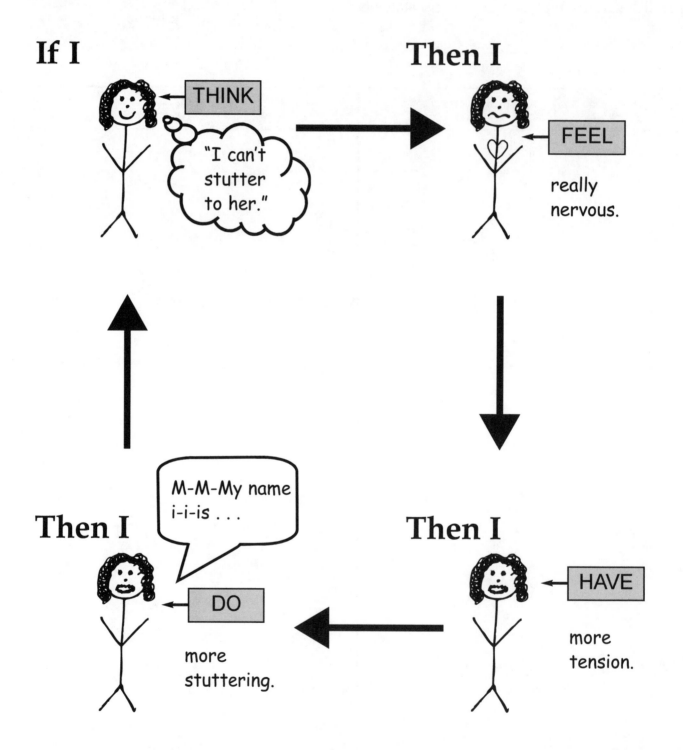

This illustration demonstrates the positive effects of accepting stuttering. Here, Angela discovers the cause and effect of changing her thinking about stuttering.

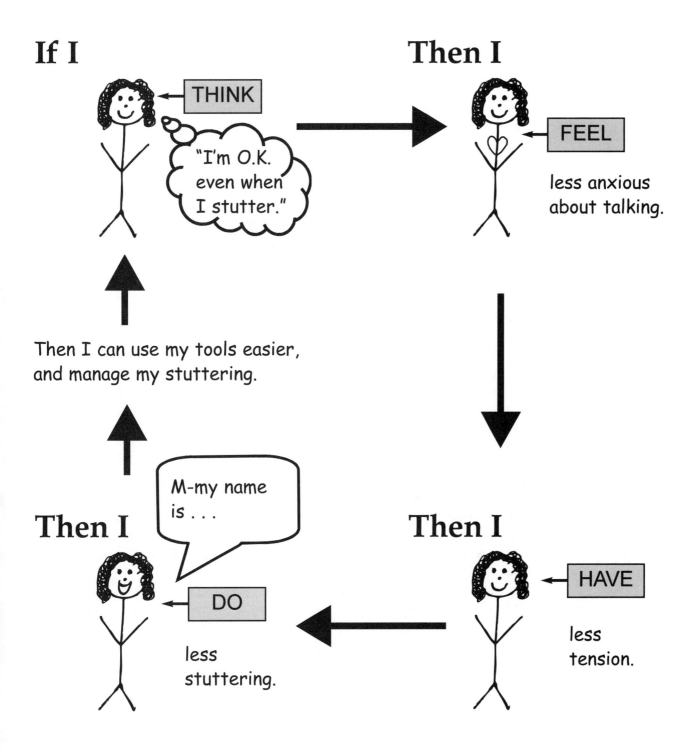

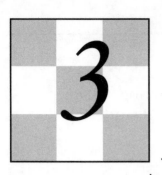

How Do I Know If He Needs Treatment?

When we ask clinicians about their goals for a diagnostic evaluation, they often tell us that the main question they are seeking to answer is whether or not the child is stuttering. Certainly, this is one important question to ask, and it is definitely one that we will need to answer during our evaluation. As we have discussed, however, children who stutter do not exhibit observable stuttering behaviors all the time, and some are quite adept at hiding their stuttering. On the other hand, the mere fact that a child stutters does not mean that he necessarily needs to be enrolled in treatment or that it is the right time for treatment. Thus, simply determining whether a child stutters during an evaluation may not give us the most meaningful or relevant information about the child's speech disorder.

For us, the key question is "should the child be enrolled in treatment right now?" All of the information we collect during a diagnostic evaluation is aimed at answering this question. In this chapter, we will discuss the factors we consider when trying to determine whether a child should be enrolled in treatment.

Getting the Big Picture

Throughout the first two chapters of this book, we highlighted the fact that there are many different (but related) factors that you can consider when working with children who stutter. Not surprisingly, this broad-based view of stuttering has strongly influenced our thinking about how to determine whether a child should be enrolled in treatment. Since so many factors can affect stuttering, we utilize a multi-factorial assessment protocol. We then consider all of the information we gather in preparing a comprehensive plan of treatment that is individualized for each child we see. Thus, throughout our assessment of a child who stutters, we are seeking to understand the "big picture."

Several authors have presented broad-based approaches to assessment (Conture 2001, Guitar 1998, Susca et al. 2002). Similarly, in this chapter, we present an approach to qualifying a child for treatment that is based not only on the child's production of speech disfluencies, but also on a comprehensive understanding of the impact of the stuttering disorder on the child's life.

Don't I just need to count the number of times he stutters?

Traditionally, the decision to enroll a child who stutters in treatment has been primarily or exclusively based upon the observable characteristics of the child's stuttering. (See reviews in Gordon & Luper 1992a, 1992b). We often read guidelines suggesting that children should receive treatment if they produce more than a certain number of disfluencies in a given conversational sample (e.g., 10% of words produced disfluently [Adams 1980]) or if their repetitions contain a certain number of iterations (e.g., more than three iterations, "li-li-li-li-like this" [Yairi & Lewis 1984]). To be sure, understanding the nature of the child's stuttering contributes to the overall understanding of the child's communication difficulties, but it is not the whole picture (Zebrowski & Conture 1997).

Once you recognize that stuttering involves much more than just speech disfluencies, you may begin to wonder whether measuring the surface stuttering behaviors can adequately tell you whether the child needs treatment. Furthermore, once you take into account factors such as the variability of stuttering and the possibility that a child may be using avoidance strategies to hide stuttering, you can see that guidelines based on the percentage of disfluencies are inadequate for documenting the true impact of stuttering on a child's ability to communicate. (Indeed, as we will discuss later in this chapter, these guidelines are also not consistent with the federal laws governing the provision of speech and language treatment to children in school settings.) If you want to make a more appropriate decision about whether a child should be enrolled in treatment—one that best positions the child for achieving success in treatment—you need more information. You need to understand the whole child and the effect the stuttering has on that child's life.

Are there any tests I can use?

We are often asked which tests we use to document how much a child stutters. By now, you will recognize that we feel strongly about the importance of taking a broad perspective when working with school-age children who stutter. Because every child who stutters is different, and because every child reacts differently to his experiences with stuttering, it is difficult for any single test or measure to capture all relevant aspects of a child's stuttering disorder. Nevertheless, we also recognize that many administrators in school districts and other clinical settings are accustomed to seeing results of specific tests or protocols for documenting a child's stuttering and for establishing eligibility for treatment. Later in this chapter, we will say more about the necessity or appropriateness of these requirements with reference to current legislation. We will also review ways you can develop your own means for thoroughly documenting the nature and extent of the child's stuttering disorder via portfolio-based assessment procedures. For now, however, we will say that the answer to the question of whether there are tests you can use to document children's stuttering is "Yes, but . . ."

Interpreting tests

There are a number of assessment protocols that can be used to document children's stuttering behaviors. Perhaps the most widely used example is the *Stuttering Severity Instrument* (SSI-3, Riley 1994) or the *Iowa Scale for Measuring the Severity of Stuttering* (Johnson et al. 1963). A number of other "standard" assessment procedures are also available (Gordon & Luper 1992a). A primary difficulty with such measures is that they generally combine all of the separate observations the clinician has made into a single label or number representing the overall stuttering severity. Thus, even though such measures by themselves provide an index of the child's stuttering severity that can be used for comparisons over time or with other children, a considerable amount of detail is lost when the numbers are scaled or collapsed across behaviors. For example, as shown in Table 3.1 on the next page, one child may score a value of 20 on a given severity test because he exhibits frequent repetitions with minimal tension, while another child may score a value of 20 on the same test because he exhibits more noticeable physical tension but fewer disfluencies. If only the severity index is considered, then the potentially important differences in the two children's stuttering behaviors would not be appreciated. *Therefore, any severity label should be accompanied by a more detailed description of the child's actual speaking and stuttering patterns.*

Furthermore, most stuttering tests focus primarily on the observable characteristics of speech, such as the frequency and type of disfluencies or the amount of visible tension and struggle the child exhibits during those disfluencies. As we have described previously, these speech behaviors constitute only a part of the overall stuttering disorder. Therefore, you need to be cautious when using such tests to make certain that you do not limit your evaluation to include only those areas identified on the stuttering test you have selected.

As you develop a broader perspective about stuttering, you will see the need to observe and document the many other aspects of the child's overall experience of stuttering. As described in more detail on the following pages, you can do this by collecting information about factors such as the child's use of avoidance strategies, the child's self-reported feelings about his or her speaking difficulties, and other factors that reflect the consequences of stuttering. When used in conjunction with standard stuttering tests, such supplemental measures can help you place stuttering severity ratings and scores from stuttering tests into the proper perspectives.

Once upon a **t-t-time**. . .	Once upon a time. . .
there was a **d-d-dinosaur** named Hubert.	there was a dinosaur named **Hhhhhhubert**.
Hubert was a Tyrannosaurus **R-r-rex**,	Hubert was a Tyrannosaurus Rex,
the scariest kind of dinosaur in the **f-f-forest**.	the scariest kind of **d----inosaur** in the forest.
But, **H-hubert** was different.	But, Hubert was different.
He wasn't **s-scary** at all.	He **wwwwwwasn't** scary at all.
Hubert **l-l-liked** to make friends	Hubert liked to make friends
and play games with all the other **d-dinosaurs**.	and play **g----ames** with all the other dinosaurs.
One **d-day**, Hubert was walking through the forest,	One day, Hubert was walking through the forest,
(boom, boom, boom)	(boom, boom, boom)
when he **m-m-met** two little girls!	when he **mmmmmet** two little girls!
Hubert was very **sur-surprised**,	Hubert was very surprised,
b-b-because he had never seen humans before.	because he had **nnnnnever** seen humans before.
He thought to himself. . .	He thought to himself. . .
"What **k-k-kind** of **d-dinosaur** is that?"	"What kind of dinosaur is that?"
He decided to **g-go** over and say hello,	He decided to go over and **sssssay** hello,
to see if he could **m-make** some new friends.	to see if he could make some new friends.

Total sample size:	100 words	Total sample size:	100 words
Total number of disfluencies:	16	Total number of disfluencies:	7
Frequency of disfluency:	16%	Frequency of disfluency:	7%
Most common disfluency type:	Repetition	Most common disfluency type:	Prolongation
Longest duration of disfluencies:	.5 seconds	Longest duration of disfluencies:	1.5 seconds
Degree of physical tension:	Very minimal	Degree of physical tension:	Mild but noticeable
Secondary behaviors:	None	Secondary behaviors:	Some eye blinks

Possible SSI-3 score: 20	Possible SSI-3 score: 20

Table 3.1   *Hypothetical speech samples from two children exhibiting different stuttering patterns but identical severity ratings.*

Stuttering—and stuttering severity—can vary

Throughout the first part of this book, we have emphasized the fact that stuttering is a highly variable disorder. Not surprisingly, this variability affects every aspect of our interaction with children, including the diagnostic evaluation and our assessment of stuttering severity. For example, if we happen to conduct our evaluation on a day when the child is particularly fluent (or disfluent), or if we select a task that evokes more or less disfluency, then our evaluation may not be representative of the child's true stuttering patterns. Therefore, we need to be cautious about over-interpreting results from stuttering tests that are based on only a few observations of the child's speech in a restricted set of situations. This is particularly relevant when you are considering eligibility criteria that may require a specific level of stuttering for entering or exiting therapy.

So what does a severity rating really tell us?

Given all of the concerns we have just raised about the use of severity measures, you might wonder if there is any value to assessing stuttering through standardized tests. We believe that there is, provided the results are placed in the proper perspective. If you keep in mind the cautions raised above, then severity measures can be useful, for they provide a more or less objective indication of the amount and nature of stuttering behaviors a student is exhibiting at a particular point in time and in a particular setting. Thus, by combining standard severity ratings with measures of the overall stuttering disorder, you can meaningfully document not only the child's status at the time of the diagnostic evaluation, but also the child's progress as he moves through therapy.

What information *do* I need to gather?

When assessing children who stutter, try to consider the child's entire communication experience, including the surface stuttering behaviors; the child's feelings, emotions, and thoughts about stuttering; the influence of the environment on the child's communication patterns; the difficulties the child may have when speaking in everyday situations; and the child's overall ability to communicate successfully. At first glance, this may seem to be too involved or more time-consuming than the quick severity measures you may be accustomed to. Nevertheless, we believe that the time is well spent. In addition to gaining necessary information about the nature of the child's stuttering disorder, a thorough assessment of the entire stuttering disorder gives you the opportunity to truly "get to know" your young clients and develop the trusting relationship you will need to help children achieve optimal success in therapy. An overview of the information gathered during a complete diagnostic evaluation for school-age children who stutter is presented in Table 3.2 on the next page. In the next sections, we will provide a more detailed explanation of the information we collect during the assessment, organized in terms of four basic questions we ask when planning our evaluation:

1. Where did the child come from?
2. Where has the child been?
3. Where is the child now?
4. Where is the child going?

Where Did the Child Come From? *(Referral Information)*

The first questions to consider have to do with who referred the child for services and why.

a. If the child transferred from another school or clinician, you will want to gather more information about his past history of therapy, including the goals that were addressed, the techniques that were used, the way he felt about therapy, his level of participation in treatment, and the successes he felt he achieved.

b. If the child was referred by a parent, you will want to gather more information about the reason for the referral, including the nature of the parent's concerns, what the parent has done to help the child in the past, and the parent's goals for therapy.

c. If the child was referred by a teacher, you will want more information about how the child's speech concerns have manifested themselves in the classroom, how the teacher has handled the situation thus far, and how other children may be reacting to the child's speaking difficulties.

Knowing more about why the child was referred will help guide your evaluation of his current situations and needs in therapy. This information can be collected through brief interviews or questionnaires completed by family members, teachers, or past clinicians, as appropriate.

55

Initial Contact

>Pre-referral
>Screening/Informal Observation
>Determination of Evaluation Domains
>Referral

In-Depth Evaluation

>Thorough Case History
>>Previous Therapy
>>Speech and Language Development
>>Significant Medical History
>>Past Academic Performance & Social History
>Assessment of Speech Fluency
>>Observable Characteristics of Stuttering
>>>(frequency, duration, type, severity of disfluency)
>>Related Behaviors (tension, struggle)
>Assessment of the Child's Reactions to Stuttering
>>Beliefs About Stuttering
>>Feelings About Stuttering and Self
>>Avoidance or Struggle Behaviors
>Assessment of Speech and Language
>>Vocabulary
>>Word Retrieval
>>Syntax
>>Oral Motor Skills
>>Speech Sound Development (articulation/phonology)
>>Voice
>Assessment of Other People's Reactions to Stuttering
>>Parents and Family
>>Teachers
>>Peers

Presentation of Results

>Evaluation of Findings
>Preparation of Report
>Conference
>>Eligibility Determination (if appropriate)
>>Development of Service Plan

Initiation of Treatment

Table 3.2   *Overview of the information gathered during a complete diagnostic evaluation for school-age children who stutter.*

The goal of gathering these types of information is to understand the specific reason that the child has been referred so you can tailor your evaluation and treatment recommendations to meet the unique needs of the child's situation.

Where Has the Child Been? (Case History)

After gathering this initial referral information, we begin to collect additional background details so we will have a more thorough understanding of where the child has been. This is generally done through a case history form, interviews with relevant people in the child's environment, and, depending upon the child's age, an interview with the child himself. We also need to document the information we have gathered through the pre-referral process.

In Appendix 3A (pages 90–93), Appendix 3C (pages 98–99), and Appendix 3E (pages 102–103), we have included forms that parents and children can fill out to provide necessary background data. We have also included some examples of forms that were completed by our own clients to demonstrate how this information is helpful in developing a plan of therapy (Appendix 3B, pages 94–97; Appendix 3D, pages 100–101; and Appendix 3F, pages 104–105). The *Stuttering Case History* form (Appendix 3A) is used to gather basic information from the parents about the child's general health status, academic performance, and social development, as well as a general description of the child's speech and stuttering. The *Parent Perceptions* form (Appendix 3C) helps parents or caregivers provide information that will help you develop the child's treatment plan, such as the emotional or cognitive reactions that the child and the people in his environment have had to stuttering, the child's use of strategies that might help or hinder his communication, and the parents' goals for therapy. Finally, the *Previous Therapy History* form (Appendix 3E) helps the child provide detailed information about any therapy he may have received prior to being referred to you. The information gained from these questionnaires not only will help you to understand the child's prior history of stuttering, it will also help you determine the type of information you will need to gather during the evaluation so you have a thorough understanding of the child's prior experiences with stuttering and stuttering therapy.

Where Is the Child Now? (Assessment)

Regardless of the child's prior experiences in or out of therapy, *the most important information influencing your decision about whether to recommend therapy is what the child is **currently** experiencing*. Thus, you need to gather information about the child's daily experiences with stuttering and communication. In the following pages, we will outline the details of a diagnostic evaluation, including information about the child's observable stuttering behaviors, the child's reactions to stuttering, the possible effect of the child's speech and language abilities on stuttering, and the impact of the child's environment on his experience of the stuttering disorder. In keeping with our general approach of organizing clinical interaction in terms of questions and answers, these sections will be presented in the form of the questions we ask ourselves during a diagnostic evaluation.

What is the nature of the child's stuttering behaviors?

Children can exhibit a variety of different types of disfluencies in their speech. Of course, not all of those disfluencies represent moments of "stuttering." All speakers produce disfluencies when speaking—disfluency is simply a normal part of the process of producing speech. Still, there is much we can learn about children's speech and stuttering by examining the different types of disfluencies they exhibit in their speech (Ambrose & Yairi 1999; Conture 2001; Curlee 1993; Yairi & Lewis 1984; Yaruss, LaSalle, et al. 1998).

In most speakers, disfluencies represent instances when speakers have, for some reason, experienced difficulty saying what they wanted to say. Perhaps they have forgotten the specific word they wanted to use, or perhaps they realized that the word or phrase was not coming out exactly the way they wanted it to—the exact reasons for disfluencies are not always clear. When speakers experience these types of momentary disruptions in speech, the disfluencies are sometimes referred to as "normal" or "nonstuttered" disfluencies. These disfluencies can take the form of:

- repetitions of words (e.g., "like-like this") or phrases (e.g., "like this—like this")
- revisions (when a speaker starts out saying one thing and then interrupts to say something else; "like thi—like that")
- interjections (e.g., "um," "uh," "you know," "like")
- long pauses or hesitations

Of course, these are not the only types of disruptions children can exhibit in their speech. Other disfluencies—the types more commonly referred to as "stuttered" or "stutter-like" disfluencies (Yairi 1996)—represent moments when the speaker knows exactly what he wants to say, but for some reason, is having difficulty actually saying it. Many times, people who stutter report a feeling of "losing control" of their speech mechanisms during stuttering, since they feel that they cannot control their mouths or voices the same way they do when they are speaking fluently (Perkins 1990).

Interestingly, these "stuttered" disfluencies generally involve interruptions *within* the word unit, as opposed to between words, which is more often the case with normal disfluencies (Conture 2001; Yaruss, LaSalle, et al. 1998). Thus, a child may exhibit a repetition of a whole word or phrase as described on the previous page, and this is generally considered to be a normal disfluency. If the repetition involves only a part of the word (a sound or syllable repetition, "li- like this"), it is generally considered to be a "stuttered" disfluency. Other types of stuttered disfluencies include *sound prolongations* ("llllllike this") and *blocks*, or moments when the child cannot seem to produce any sound at all ("l---ike this"). Regardless of the specific type of disfluency that is observed, all of these "stuttered" disfluencies represent moments when the speaker cannot say what he wants to say. Figure 3.1 on the next page gives examples of "normal" and "stuttered" disfluencies and demonstrates the presumed relationship between the various disfluency types.

Differences between disfluency types

There are three important points to remember about the differences between the disfluencies exhibited by children who stutter and those exhibited by children who do not stutter. First, all speakers—even children who do not stutter—can exhibit all of the different types of disfluencies in their speech. Thus, the presence of so-called "stuttered" disfluencies does not by itself indicate that a child is stuttering (Johnson & Associates 1959). Of course, the reverse is also true: a stretch of speech that does not contain any disfluencies does not, by itself, indicate that a child is not at risk for stuttering. The differences between children who stutter and children who do not stutter are not always seen in the types of disfluencies, but rather in the relative frequency of the different types of disfluencies (Conture 2001). Children who do not stutter tend to produce more of the normal types of disfluencies (phrase repetitions, revisions, interjections), while children who do

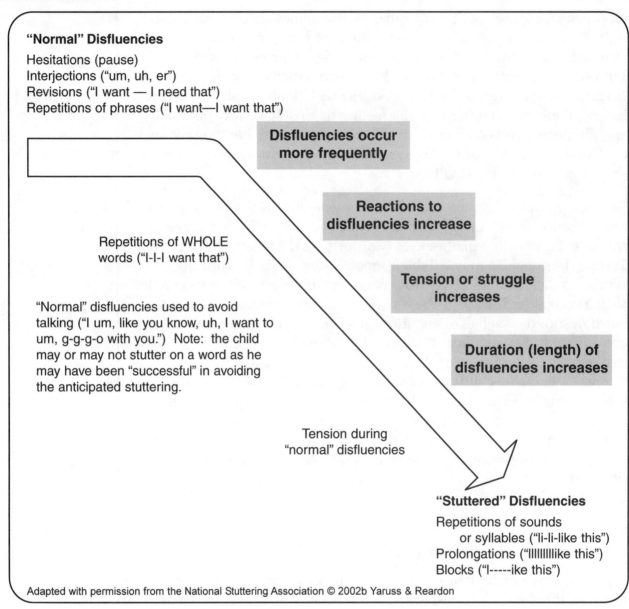

"Normal" Disfluencies

Hesitations (pause)
Interjections ("um, uh, er")
Revisions ("I want — I need that")
Repetitions of phrases ("I want—I want that")

Repetitions of WHOLE
words ("I-I-I want that")

"Normal" disfluencies used to avoid
talking ("I um, like you know, uh, I want to
um, g-g-g-o with you.") Note: the child
may or may not stutter on a word as he
may have been "successful" in avoiding
the anticipated stuttering.

Tension during
"normal" disfluencies

**Disfluencies occur
more frequently**

**Reactions to
disfluencies increase**

**Tension or struggle
increases**

**Duration (length) of
disfluencies increases**

"Stuttered" Disfluencies

Repetitions of sounds
or syllables ("li-li-like this")
Prolongations ("Illlllllike this")
Blocks ("I-----ike this")

Adapted with permission from the National Stuttering Association © 2002b Yaruss & Reardon

Figure 3.1 *Different types of speech disfluencies*

stutter tend to produce more of the stuttered types of disfluencies
(sound/syllable repetitions, prolongations, blocks). Children who
stutter may also produce a high frequency of so-called normal
disfluencies.

The second important point is the fact that normal disfluencies may
actually serve to hide or mask instances when a child is experiencing
a moment of real stuttering under the surface (Manning 2001). In
other words, a child may use interjections or phrase repetitions to
postpone or change a word he thought he was about to stutter on.
For example, when a child says "I want the... uh... the... uh... uh...

the book," it is possible that the repetition of the word *the* and the interjection of *uh* may have been used to postpone production of the word *book* if the child thought he might stutter on *book*. Thus, although so-called "normal" disfluencies often indicate typical disruptions in the children's speech patterns (e.g., the child is thinking about what he wants to say), they may also indicate that stuttering is occurring under the surface. For this reason, it may be difficult, if not impossible, for you to determine exactly how many times a child truly stutters during a speech sample.

The third important point about differences between normal disfluency and stuttered disfluencies is that all of these different disfluency types can be accompanied by physical tension or struggle behaviors which indicate that the child is having difficulty speaking. These struggle behaviors—which are perhaps the most observable or noticeable aspect of stuttering—are far more likely to be seen in children who stutter than in children who do not stutter. Again, though, a child who is adept at hiding his stuttering may not exhibit any obvious tension during his apparently normal disfluencies, so the lack of struggle does not necessarily indicate that a child is not experiencing stuttering.

"Normal" and "Stuttered" Disfluencies

All children produce all different types of disfluencies. Both stuttering and normally fluent children exhibit both "stuttered" and "normal" disfluencies in their speech.

Not all "normal" disfluencies are normal. Sometimes, "normal" disfluencies may hide or mask instances when a child is experiencing a moment of real stuttering under the surface.

All types of disfluencies may be accompanied by physical tension or struggle. This physical tension is far more likely to be seen in children who stutter.

Obtaining representative samples

Regardless of the problems inherent in differentiating stuttered and normal disfluencies, it is still important to document the amount of disfluency we see in a child's speech. In doing so, we try to be mindful of the potential pitfalls highlighted above so we can obtain the most accurate representation we can of a child's stuttering during a particular speaking situation at a given point in time.

We have long been interested in researching the methods different clinicians use for measuring stuttering (e.g., Yaruss 1997a, b, 1998b, 2000; Yaruss et al. 1998). Through these studies and our clinical practice, we have seen clinicians use many different techniques for counting stuttering events, from simply making marks on a sheet of paper to indicate the number of times a child stutters to using a specialized form for counting disfluencies to completing a detailed verbatim transcript of a child's speech based on repeated examination of an audiotaped or videotaped speech sample. Similarly, we know some clinicians who count the number of words stuttered and others who count the number of syllables stuttered; some who use speech samples of 100 words (or syllables) and others who are not satisfied with less than 500. There are some clinicians who collect data in the therapy room and some who collect data in the classroom. And there are some clinicians who mark all disfluencies the child produces and others who mark only those disfluencies they judge to be stuttered.

Example Speaking Situations, Speaking Tasks, and Conversational Partners

Speaking Settings
classroom
clinic
cafeteria
hallway
playground

Speaking Tasks
conversation (dialogue)
reading
describing a simple or complex picture
retelling a familiar story or recent experience (e.g., vacation)
retelling a less familiar story or describing a lesson from class

Conversational Partners
peers
teachers
siblings
parents or other family members
unfamiliar listeners/strangers

Regardless of the specific decisions clinicians make about these details, there are some guidelines that should be kept in mind to support the accurate interpretation of the frequency count. First of all, you will need to collect data from more than one speaking situation if you wish to understand the variability of a child's stuttering (e.g., Costello & Ingham 1984, Gregory & Hill 1999, Yaruss 1997a). Because every child is different, the specific situations you examine will differ from child to child. Indeed, research has shown that there is no single situation that evokes either more stuttering or more fluency from all children.

Possibilities for different speaking situations include the child's classroom, the playground, the cafeteria or lunchroom, the therapy room, and home samples that the family can provide. You can also consider different speaking tasks, such as producing a narrative, retelling a story, and engaging in conversation with you, a parent, or a peer. In other words, try to gain a representative indication of the child's stuttering in different situations by varying the settings in which the child is speaking, the speaking task the child is performing, and the conversational partners with whom the child is speaking. Examples of some situations we have used are listed in the box on the previous page.

Of course, we cannot observe every child in all of the situations described in the box. We use the information obtained from the interview and case history forms to determine which situations appear to be most relevant for each individual child, then we try to obtain representative samples from an appropriate subset of those situations. Generally, we find that two to three situations are sufficient, if they are selected carefully. We try not to spend too much of our assessment time focusing on the measure of frequency of stuttering, for it is only one aspect of the stuttering disorder that needs to be addressed in an evaluation.

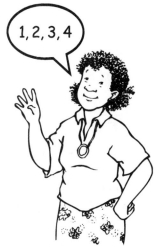

The assessment of different speaking situations allows you to examine the factors that may affect the child's speech. Factors to consider include linguistic complexity, number and nature of conversational partners, location, and other issues such as excitement level, familiarity of the material being discussed, whether the child is talking about objects or events that are present or distant (i.e., referential language), etc. You also gain useful information about speaking situations you may need to address with the child in treatment.

A second aspect of frequency counts that must be considered is the size of the speech samples upon which counts are based. This is relevant for two reasons.

1. If the samples are too small, they will not truly represent the children's speech fluency in different situations. We prefer samples of at least 200 to 300 words (or syllables) in each situation, though the larger the samples, the more representative the data (Conture 2001, Yairi 1997).

2. It is also important to report the size of the sample upon which the observations are based. We often see reports indicating that a child exhibited, "10 stutters" during an evaluation, or that he stuttered

on "10 sentences." Unfortunately, without knowing the size of the sample, we cannot interpret such statements or compare them to other measures. More meaningful is a statement that says that the child exhibited "10 sound repetitions in a sample of 500 words" (i.e., stuttering on 2% of the words in the sample) (Conture 2001).

Even though frequency counts can only give us a snapshot of a constantly varying behavior, the measures we make should still be as accurate as possible. Thus, an indication of the frequency of disfluencies (number of disfluencies per number of words) is more useful than an indication of the raw number of disfluencies.

Much has been written about the inaccuracy of frequency counts, and, indeed, research has demonstrated that different clinicians do not generally achieve the same results when analyzing children's speech samples (Cordes 1994, Cordes & Ingham 1994a). This means that it can be difficult to use frequency counts when comparing different children, or the same children over time. Still, research has also demonstrated that a clinician's reliability in counting stuttering can be increased dramatically through practice (Costello & Hurst 1981). We have definitely found this to be true in our own work. We encourage you to invest a little bit of time practicing frequency counts. At first, it may seem very difficult, but over time it will become faster, easier, and more reliable (Yaruss 1998b).

Guidelines for Obtaining Representative Samples

1. *Remember that frequency counts are just a snapshot.* Because observable stuttering behaviors vary depending upon the speaking task, the setting, and the conversational partner, frequency counts only represent a child's speech at a single point in time in a specific situation.

2. *Collect data from more than one sample.* To obtain a representative picture of a child's fluency, it will be necessary to collect speech samples in a variety of situations.

3. *Remember individual variability.* The specific factors that affect the speech of a given child will not be the same as those that affect the speech of another child.

4. *Collect large enough samples.* If the speech sample is too small, it will not truly represent the child's speech in that situation.

5. *Practice to develop reliability.* Research has shown that the reliability of stuttering counts improve through practice. Without this practice, frequency counts may not accurately represent a child's speech.

As we have stated, there are many different ways to count stuttering events, and it does not appear that any one way is better than the others. You can count words or syllables, 100-word or 500-word samples, and in "real-time" or from a videotape. Research seems to suggest that it doesn't really matter which decisions you make about the aspects of measurement (Yaruss 1997b, 1998b, 2000; Yaruss, Max, et al. 1998). What does matter is that you know *why* you are selecting a particular measurement strategy, and that you *document* the measurement strategies you use so other clinicians will be able to make use of the data in a meaningful way.

So how do we measure stuttering frequency?

Even with all the concerns stated above, it is still possible to obtain meaningful counts of children's speech disfluencies. Learning to calculate the frequency of stuttering takes some time and effort, but the process is generally straightforward.

In essence, to determine a child's average frequency of stuttering, we observe a child speaking in different situations and keep track of how many times the child produces disfluencies of various types. This can either be done in real-time or from a videotape, though we prefer and recommend videotape, as *we do not complete our frequency count sheets while we are actually engaged in conversation with the child.*

To facilitate our analysis, we use a count sheet, such as the one shown in Figure 3.2. (A full-size form can be found in Appendix 3G, page 106). The count sheet we use has four sections with 100 spaces each, representing the words (or syllables) the child produces. We prefer to collect between 200- and 400-word samples in each situation we observe, so we may use more than one count sheet each time we are measuring a child's stuttering frequency.

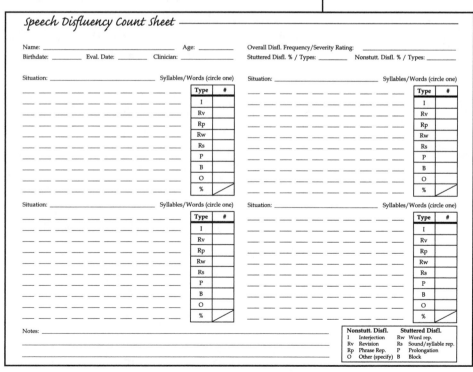

Figure 3.2 (A full-size form can be found in Appendix 3G, page 106.)

For each word that we perceive to be fluent, we mark a dash or a dot on the form in the space representing that word. If the child produces a disfluency, then we write an abbreviation indicating the type of disfluency in the appropriate space. Thus, if the child produces an interjection ("um," "uh"), we can mark an "I" in the space representing that word, and if the child exhibits a sound or syllable repetition ("li-like this"), we can use the mark "SSR" for "sound/syllable repetition" (Conture 2001) or "Rs" (for "repetition of a syllable") (Gregory & Hill 1999). The abbreviations we typically use are similar to those used by other authors (See review in Yaruss 1997b). They are listed in the key on the form.

We then calculate the frequency of disfluencies for each set of 100 words by simply counting up the total number of disfluencies in each section (Conture 2001, Yaruss 1998b). We can also calculate the relative frequency of the different types of disfluencies the child has produced in the sample by counting up the number of each type of disfluency (e.g., interjections, sound/syllable repetitions, phrase repetitions) that the child exhibited in each 100-word (or syllable) section. We then write that number in the tally section that accompanies each block of 100 words. This helps us obtain the profile of disfluency types that are most often produced by that child (Yaruss et al. 1998).

In summary, we can use the count sheet to quickly gather relevant information about the surface characteristics of a child's stuttering. An example of a completed count sheet is included in Appendix 3H, page 107. Keep in mind that the procedures we have just described represent just one way of obtaining stuttering frequency counts. Other clinicians may make different decisions about how to measure the observable features of stuttering (e.g., Campbell & Hill 1987, Cordes & Ingham 1994b). The specific decisions a clinician makes about how to gather this information (e.g., words vs. syllables, sample size) are less important than the reliability of the measures. This reliability can be increased dramatically if you practice and if you carefully document your measures of the observable characteristics of the stuttering disorder. This information is then placed in context with the rest of the diagnostic evaluation as we attempt to understand the true impact of stuttering on the child's life.

In addition to calculating the frequency of various types of disfluencies, we can also obtain additional information about the surface characteristics of the child's stuttering. Examples of such measures include the *duration* of disfluencies (Zebrowski 1991, 1994) and the number of iterations in repetitions (Throneburg & Yairi 1994, Yairi & Lewis 1984). Some clinicians have suggested that the duration of disfluencies can be calculated using a stopwatch; however, we do not prefer to have the child see or hear us clicking the button on the stopwatch while he is trying to communicate. As with the frequency counts, we prefer to be engaged in conversation with the child rather than diverting our attention to data collection. Furthermore, we have found that it is often sufficient simply to estimate the average duration of the child's disfluencies (by counting seconds in our heads). If a more precise calculation is necessary, we can always videotape the conversation and complete our counts and measures afterwards.

Regardless of the method used for measuring duration, longer disfluencies generally indicate that the child is experiencing more tension or struggle during stuttering. Thus, a more direct measure of the tension and struggle a child exhibits may be more useful. This can best be obtained through a detailed narrative description of the child's speech behaviors during stuttering. Specific characteristics to consider include eye blinks; observable tension in the lips, tongue, throat, and larynx; movements of the head and neck; and even movements in other parts of the body. (Note that this information is incorporated into measures such as the *Stuttering Severity Index* (SSI) and the Iowa scale; however, it is combined with measures of other aspects of stuttering, so specific data about the child's tension and struggle can easily be lost or overlooked.)

Of course, not all stuttering events are the same. As we watch a child speaking and stuttering, however, we are generally able to get a sense for the pattern of disfluencies that he typically exhibits. In other words, although children stutter differently from one another, there are often similarities within an individual child in terms of the disfluency pattern he exhibits. Some children tend to produce more prolongations and others tend to produce more repetitions, some tend to blink their eyes while others tend to exhibit tension in their lips. By examining these patterns and describing them in detail on our count sheet, we can develop a useful record of the nature of the child's stuttering events.

What are the child's beliefs and feelings?

Among the areas that have historically been most difficult to assess are the beliefs and feelings a child may have about his speech and stuttering. A child's feelings about his speech—and about himself—can play an important role in determining the nature of his stuttering disorder and, importantly, the progress he will make in therapy (Manning 2001).

In fact, a child's reactions to stuttering are probably the most critical factors influencing his ability to manage stuttering over the long term.

Talking with children about their feelings

Many times, clinicians tell us that they are uncomfortable talking with children about their feelings. We recognize, of course, that most SLPs do not have training in counseling methods, so their discomfort is understandable. Still, we feel that clinicians do not necessarily need to have an extensive background in psychology to help most children who stutter evaluate and process their feelings about their speech. Children open up to people who relate to them, validate their feelings, and create an atmosphere of acceptance and openness. As SLPs, we can do our best work by providing children with a safe, trusted environment where they can explore how they feel about themselves and their speech. We will provide more details about specific counseling strategies that are used in treatment for school-age children who stutter in the next two chapters. For the present, however, it is important to recognize that you *can* and *should* give children the opportunity to express their feelings about stuttering during the diagnostic evaluation and later, during treatment.

Developing counseling skills

Numerous resources are available for helping you develop counseling skills. Several examples can be found in the list of resources in Appendix 2A, pages 45–46. The strategies described in these resources can be quite useful for helping you learn to assess and deal with the beliefs and feelings of children who stutter, as well as those of the parents and other significant individuals in a child's environment.

Depending upon the clinical setting in which you work, you may be able to develop partnerships with many other helpful professionals, such as social workers and school counselors or psychologists. Indeed, there are many disciplines that devote all of their research, energies, and resources to expanding our understanding of children's feelings. These resources can provide you with additional strategies for addressing a child's reactions to stuttering and their influence on a child's self-esteem and communication skills. Thus, you are not alone in helping children deal with their feelings, and you can draw upon your colleagues and other resources as you work to develop your own counseling skills. The time you invest in learning how to relate to children more effectively will not only serve the children who stutter, it will also enhance your clinical effectiveness with all of the children with whom you work.

Assessing children's feelings about stuttering

The most straightforward way to gather information about a child's feelings and perceptions about his stuttering is by talking directly with the child. First of all, you need to be aware of the child's level of comfort when talking about stuttering. Depending upon the child's age and awareness of stuttering, you may choose to begin with quiet play activities that allow you to engage in conversations about his interests, friends, and eventually, his communication. Strive to interact with the child on a level that allows him to see that you are someone he can trust. This trust makes it easier for the child to tell you things about his speech that he may not have shared with anyone else. The following are examples of the types of information you can gather during a child interview.

- How concerned does the child seem to be about his speech?
- How does the child feel about past therapy experiences?
- Does the child seem to be interested in speech therapy at the present time?
- What does the child know about stuttering?
- How accurate are the child's beliefs about stuttering?
- What does the child call his speaking difficulty?
- How accurately can the child describe the speech behaviors he exhibits?
- What does the child do to try to prevent or minimize stuttering?
- What strategies does the child use when he is having trouble speaking?
- How does the child feel about the reactions of others?
- How does the child feel about himself as a communicator?

During the interview, you can watch the child's nonverbal reactions in addition to listening to his verbal reactions to gain an understanding of his feelings and beliefs about stuttering. In addition to the interview, you can use tests to measure a child's communication attitudes (DeNil & Brutten 1991). Unfortunately, relatively few tests are available for school-age children who stutter. Such tests can provide you with information about how a particular child may think or feel about his communication skills by gathering responses to statements such as "I have trouble speaking" or "Other people worry about my speech." These measures can be useful tools for meeting eligibility requirements and providing progress updates in school districts that require specific tests. They are not necessarily easy for children to complete because most feelings are complex and not simply "all on" or "all off." In fact, the most common answer we often receive to such standard measures is "sometimes." Fortunately, normed tests are not the only vehicle for documenting change in beliefs and feelings.

Another strategy for evaluating the beliefs and feelings of children who stutter is by using portfolio assessment procedures. Portfolio assessment involves a variety of paper-and-pencil measures that give the child the opportunity to explore and express the affective and cognitive reactions he may have to his stuttering (Chmela & Reardon 2001). We recognize that some clinicians and administrators may initially be unfamiliar or uncomfortable with these approaches because they are not standardized. Nevertheless, this approach to evaluation can provide a significant advantage over standard communication attitudes inventories because these measures can be tailored to meet the needs of each individual child. Furthermore, as we will discuss at the end of this chapter, portfolio assessment procedures are quite consistent with the evaluation strategies recommended by current legislation governing public education of children with communication disorders (e.g., IDEA).

In developing our portfolio assessment procedures, we have drawn upon several assessment strategies from other disciplines, as discussed above.

On the next page, you will find two examples of portfolio-based documentation. In the first example, Brad, age 13, used the first letters in the word *stuttering* to generate words that related to his beliefs and feelings about his speech. This activity can be done with any word a child uses to talk about his speech. In the second example, the clinician utilized a portfolio documentation strategy that involved creating a transcript of an actual conversation that took place during an initial assessment. It reflects how Kyle, age 8, describes his stuttering.

Specific Examples of Assessment Strategies

- reflective writings and drawings
- journal entries
- questionnaires
- checklists
- transcripts of conversations with the child
- documentation of behaviors (or changes in behavior) observed by the SLP, teachers, parents, or peers

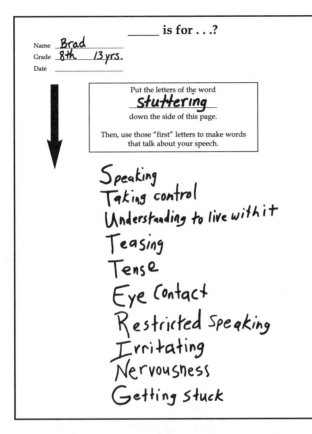

_____ is for . . .?

Name **Brad**
Grade **8th** **13 yrs.**
Date _____

Put the letters of the word
stuttering
down the side of this page.

Then, use those "first" letters to make words
that talk about your speech.

Speaking
Taking control
Understanding to live with it
Teasing
Tense
Eye Contact
Restricted speaking
Irritating
Nervousness
Getting stuck

Portfolio Documentation Sheet

Date _____
Student _**Kyle**_

Kyle and I put together a puzzle that he brought with him from the classroom. As we did this, we discussed his friends and what they liked to do after school. Then, we talked about who Kyle liked to talk to the most and what they liked to talk about.

- When I asked him if "talking was ever hard for him," Kyle said, "Yes, sometimes."
- When I asked him to tell me what that felt like, he said that it "feels like I can't get the words out and they get stuck."
- He also mentioned that "It's not bumpy or repeating, it's like I can't say it at all."

Although the purpose of portfolio assessment is to help you understand the child's affective, behavioral, and cognitive reactions to his stuttering, it is worth noting that these exercises also provide a very useful tool for helping _the child_ understand his own reactions. For this reason, we use many similar techniques in an ongoing manner throughout the treatment process to help children access their feelings about stuttering and, ultimately, learn to modify them. For now, it is important to acknowledge that it is necessary and appropriate for you to talk with a child about how he feels about his speech when attempting to determine whether he should be recommended for therapy.

What about other aspects of speech and language development?

Stuttering can certainly be affected by the child's other speech and language skills, for stuttering happens in the context of conversation (Conture 2001). As you assess the entire scope of a child's communication skills, you may find that there are phonological, articulation, oral-motor, voice, or language deficits—or strengths—that impact the child's ability to communicate freely. Because these areas are all part of the child's overall communication effectiveness, they can also influence the child's stuttering. Note that the reverse is also true, since children who stutter may not have the same speaking experiences as other children. As a result, they may not have the same opportunities to develop and hone their communication skills. A detailed explanation of general speech and language testing is outside the scope of this book, of course, but you must be prepared to assess many aspects of a child's overall communication abilities to determine whether they affect (or have been affected by) the child's stuttering.

There are a number of specific characteristics of children's speech and language development that we pay particular attention to. One such area is articulation and phonological development. Research has shown that many preschool children who stutter exhibit difficulties with speech sound production (Fosnot 1993, Louko et al. 1990, St. Louis & Hinzman 1988, Yaruss et al. 1998). Although most children's speech sound systems have resolved by the time they have reached the school-age years, it is possible that some children's speech sound difficulties may have persisted.

In addition, it has been suggested that some children who stutter may also experience subtle oral-motor difficulties (Riley & Riley 1986), so a thorough assessment of diadochokinetic abilities may also be indicated. Difficulties with intelligibility and correct speech sound production can pose a particular difficulty for children who may already be experiencing frustration with their speaking abilities. Facing situations where other people have difficulty understanding them can significantly complicate matters for children who stutter. As we discuss in the next chapter, an open, honest, and supportive assessment of a child's speaking abilities can help a child learn to accept his speech so he can approach the task of communication without the negative emotions that plague so many children who stutter.

Of course, children who are experiencing difficulties with expressive or receptive language will need additional support and treatment. Do not overlook the possible impact the language concerns may have on the child's ability to communicate freely and effectively. Finally, one other component of language development that may be relevant for school-age children who stutter is lexical access or "word-finding." Although there is no conclusive research on the topic, it has been suggested that some children who stutter may have difficulty with this component of language formulation (Gregory & Hill 1999). It may, therefore, be helpful to assess word-finding abilities in children who stutter if a screening suggests that there might be a difficulty in this area. The same is true for narrative abilities and storytelling. In general, it seems sensible to assess any aspect of speech or language development that appears to affect a child's stuttering (as determined through the examination of different speaking tasks and situations) so that you can determine if supplemental treatment in these areas might support the child's ability to communicate freely and effectively.

What is the impact of the environment?

As we discuss in Chapter 6, children do not stutter "in a vacuum." In other words, children affect—and are affected by—the environments in which they live. Thus, if you wish to develop a thorough understanding of the overall impact of stuttering on the child's life, you also need to ask questions about the situations in which the child lives. Several examples of areas we consider are listed below. Of course, it is impossible to develop a complete list of questions that might be relevant for a particular child; however, we are able to use the information gathered in other portions of the assessment to guide our data collection.

- What do people in the child's environment know about stuttering in general?
- How do significant individuals in the child's environment feel about the child who stutters or about his stuttering?
- What advice do family members or friends provide the child about how to control stuttering?
- What are the family's beliefs and feelings about the goals of stuttering therapy?
- How does the family define successful treatment?
- What is the family's opinion about prior therapy?
- What is the family's opinion about the child's past motivation in treatment?
- How involved was the family in any prior treatment?
- What have teachers or other people at school said to the child about stuttering?

You can gather much of this information using the same types of portfolio assessment procedures described on pages 70–71 and through interviews with family members, teachers, peers where necessary, and, certainly, the child himself. The overall goal of this portion of the evaluation process is to determine if the child or any of the important people in his environment hold opinions or beliefs about stuttering that may affect his progress in therapy. Negative attitudes, misconceptions about the nature of the disorder, or a lack of understanding of the goals of treatment can impede a child's ability to accept stuttering and reduce his ability to manage his speech over the long term. Thus, the more you know about the child's environment, the more you can tailor your treatment to the needs of the child.

One particularly important aspect of the child's environment to consider is the school environment. The attitudes of the child's teachers and peers can have a significant impact on his ability to communicate at school. Therefore, we use portfolio assessment procedures to gather information about what people at the child's school know about stuttering, how they feel about the child who stutters, and how they have reacted to stuttering in the past. The *Teacher Checklist – Stuttering* (Appendix 3I, pages 108–110) helps teachers provide information about how the child's stuttering may affect his participation in classroom activities. This form also gathers information about how stuttering may affect a child's interactions with peers in the classroom setting. A sample *Teacher Checklist – Stuttering* can be found in Appendix 3J, pages 111–113. The *My Thoughts About School* form (Appendix 3K, page 114) gives the child an opportunity to give his own perspective about his experiences in the school setting. You can use this information, combined with information the child provides, to determine whether you need to address any issues the child may be facing at school.

What else do I need to know?

Every child is different from every other child, and every child who stutters is different from every other child who stutters. Therefore, it is difficult for any standard assessment protocol to address all of the important aspects of stuttering for any one particular child. Furthermore, because stuttering affects so many aspects of a child's life, you do not always know when you have assessed everything that is relevant for a particular child. Our answer is to design the most comprehensive evaluation you can so you can prepare yourself to develop the most targeted treatment program you can. You also will have many more opportunities to learn about the child and his stuttering during the treatment process, so you can constantly monitor the child's observable stuttering behaviors, his affective and cognitive reactions to stuttering, his speech and language abilities, and environmental reactions to determine whether you will need to make modifications to the treatment program.

Where Is the Child Going?
(Treatment Recommendations)

By the time you have completed the diagnostic evaluation, you will have gathered a significant amount of information about the child's speaking abilities, communication patterns, personality, and degree of concern about stuttering. You will have also learned about the impact of the child's environment, and you will have begun to develop a rapport with the child and several key individuals in the child's life. Together, these and other factors will help you understand the impact of stuttering on the child's ability to participate in academic and social activities.

The next challenge is to integrate this information to obtain an overall picture of the child and his needs in therapy. To help you do this, and to help you communicate your findings to other relevant individuals, you might use a summary form such as the *Overall Evaluation Summary* (Appendix 3L, page 115).

As you look at summary forms from different children, you can see that each child exhibits a different stuttering pattern and has different needs for therapy. As we will discuss in the next chapter, you can build a truly individualized therapy approach for every child you see based on the information you have gathered during the diagnostic evaluation. First, however, you must take the information gathered during the diagnostic evaluation and determine whether you want to refer the child for treatment.

When is it "bad" enough for therapy?

When you make recommendations about whether a child should be enrolled in therapy, the question to ask yourself is not whether the child is stuttering; that much is generally obvious, unless the child is quite adept at hiding his stuttering. The question is also not whether the child is stuttering at a certain prescribed level (e.g., a criterion level or cut-off for the frequency of stuttering). Instead, you need to focus on *whether the child is ready for therapy*, that is, whether he is at a point in his academic or social development so that he will be able to benefit from therapy.

There are two critical consequences of this approach to determining which children should be referred for therapy. The first is the fact that some children may be referred for treatment even if they exhibit a relatively low frequency of stuttering behaviors. If a child exhibits significant negative affective or cognitive reactions to stuttering, or if he is using avoidance or escape behaviors to prevent stuttering behaviors from being obvious to the listener, then he may be significantly in need of therapy even though he appears to stutter rarely.

Questions to Ask Ourselves When Determining Whether to Recommend Therapy

1. What factors appear to affect the child's fluency in different speaking situations?

2. Does the child exhibit physical tension during stuttering?

3. Does the child exhibit negative reactions to stuttering (e.g., fear, anxiety)?

4. Does the child try to prevent stuttering by avoiding words, sounds, or situations?

5. Does the child express a willingness to participate in therapy?

6. What were the child's experiences in past therapy?

7. How does the child feel about prior therapy experiences?

8. Does the child utilize speech therapy strategies learned in prior therapy?

9. Is the child experiencing negative consequences as a result of stuttering?

10. Is the child being teased about stuttering?

11. How is the stuttering affecting the child's life?

12. What are the child's goals for therapy?

13. Is the child's self-esteem affected by stuttering or experiences related to stuttering?

14. Does the child seem ready for therapy?

The second consequence of our approach to enrolling children in treatment is the fact that some children who stutter—even those who stutter severely—may not necessarily receive treatment. For example, if it appears that it is not the right time for them to be in therapy, or if they are not ready to benefit from therapy, then it makes little sense to force them into therapy they do not want. On the other hand, if it is apparent that they already possess tools for managing their speech and accepting stuttering, and if they have already learned to communicate effectively and feel good about themselves, then they may not need therapy *even if they still stutter.* In such cases, your role may be to help the child's family and others in his environment understand that it is okay for the child to stutter. They may not realize that continued stuttering is not simply a sign of laziness or that the child is not "using his tools." Or they may have forgotten (or they may never have been told) that stuttering is a neurophysiologic condition that affects the child's speech production; it is not simply a behavior that he can choose to do or not do. Thus, sometimes a child will stutter but still not need therapy, and you can bring about a positive change in the child's life if you can help the people in his environment understand this important fact.

What's the difference between "needing" therapy and "benefiting from" therapy?

At first glance, the distinction between "needing" therapy and "being able to benefit from" therapy may seem subtle and not particularly important. Some clinicians may believe that all school-age children who stutter should be enrolled in therapy simply because they stutter. By now, it should be clear that we view the situation somewhat differently and that we try to recommend therapy for children who *need* treatment and *can benefit* from treatment.

We can say with confidence that nearly all children who stutter can benefit from treatment. By this, we mean that there are probably aspects of acceptance of stuttering or modification of speech that nearly all children who stutter could improve. Which of us could not benefit from additional attention paid to an aspect of our life that troubles us? Still, we feel that this is different from needing therapy.

When we say that a child needs therapy, we mean that he is facing a problem in his life due to his stuttering, such as negative communication attitudes, low self-esteem, shame or embarrassment about his speech, difficulties with self-acceptance, challenges communicating effectively with others, or limitations in his ability to participate in academic or social activities. It is reasonable to say that the vast majority of children who stutter are at risk for experiencing these negative consequences; however, it is not necessarily a given. Thus, although nearly all children who stutter *could* benefit from therapy, not all children who stutter *need* therapy.

One consequence of this approach is the fact that recommending a child for therapy means that you are making a meaningful judgment about the impact of the stuttering on the child's life. Those children who are experiencing a negative impact from stuttering will be recommended for treatment, while those who are not experiencing that negative impact may not be. Again, the majority of children who stutter will indeed experience those negative consequences. Still, you should not view yourself as the "speech police" and try to "correct" or eliminate all signs of stuttering in every child you meet.

Is now the right time?

Many times, we find that children who stutter are in therapy for year after year, making little or no progress in either their abilities to use speech management strategies or in their attitudes and feelings toward stuttering. Often, these are the children who grow up believing that therapy did not work for them—and, unfortunately, they are correct. Regardless of your therapeutic philosophy or your approach to stuttering, determining the right time for therapy is a delicate balance. In our experience, different children who stutter are ready for therapy at different times in their life experiences.

In order to determine the readiness of any child, you must first understand that long-term success in therapy includes a variety of goals. At any given point in time, a child may be ready to address some treatment goals but not others. For example, a child may be ready for education about speech and stuttering even if he is not ready to explore his feelings or learn to accept some moments of stuttered speech. Another child may be unwilling to work on speech techniques but may be ready to get seriously involved in desensitization and working on attitudes regarding stuttering and communication. Yet another child might be fairly comfortable with stuttering but still want to practice techniques so his speech will be as fluent as possible in certain situations. Thus, when you are trying to determine if you should recommend a child for therapy, you need to take into account the specific goals you will be setting for the child. You will not want to set specific goals in areas where the child is not ready to make progress, though a lack of readiness in some areas does not necessarily mean a lack of readiness in other areas.

How do I gauge a child's readiness?

Unfortunately, there is no simple test or measure we can apply to gauge a child's readiness for treatment. The best tool we know of is our connection with the child and our understanding of the child's experiences with his stuttering. As we discuss in Chapter 1, and as numerous authors have emphasized, the rapport that we build with the child is one of the most critical factors determining whether or not our therapy will be successful. If you have taken the time to get to know the whole child, you will have a deeper insight and intuition into his level of readiness for the activities and concepts involved in the therapy process.

Sometimes the best therapy is no therapy

Often, the children we evaluate have been in therapy for a long time. They may feel that they have "learned it all" or that "therapy just doesn't work." If this is their opinion about treatment, then it is unlikely that they will be interested in trying more therapy with a new clinician. Of course, you will do your best to explain to them the opportunities they may face in treatment, either because they will be trying a different approach and focusing on different goals or because they are older and better able to incorporate speech changes into their lives. Nevertheless, sometimes children who have been in treatment in the past are just ready for a break. Another situation you might face is the child who is just not interested in therapy. Even if a child experiences negative consequences due to his stuttering, this does not necessarily mean that he is going to be willing to put in the time or effort involved in making changes in his speech or attitudes about stuttering.

As mentioned previously, we take a long-term view of recovery from stuttering. Recall that our overall goal for treatment is to help children learn to live successfully with their stuttering. We want to help them minimize the impact of stuttering so they can communicate freely and feel good about themselves. Because our goal is not simply to try to completely eliminate stuttering (something that does not appear to be possible for many school-age children who stutter), we feel perfectly comfortable giving children a break from therapy if they want it (a "speech vacation"), or postponing our treatment recommendation until a child is ready.

It is important to remember that the most positive changes in our lives take place when we are ready to make changes. A child who is not interested in making changes to his speech during therapy will likely

Here is an example of a *Speech Vacation Plan* developed by Paul, age 10, as he planned to take a short break from weekly speech therapy. Paul, his speech therapist, and his parents were all involved in the discussions regarding this plan. Together they discussed what their roles would be for helping to make Paul's speech vacation a positive opportunity for reflection during a time of decreased therapy activity.

Name: __Paul__   Grade: __4__

The "Paul's Excellent Adventure" Speech Vacation Plan

Where are we going? "speech break"

Who will be going? Mrs. Nina, dad, mom, Paul

Plans for everyone - [Itineraries]

① Paul's role -
  • Using Tools + raise hand more often in school.
② Mom and Dad's role -
  • Helping Paul if they see him getting stuck in avoidance
  • Call Mrs. Nina to touch base
  • get calendar for Paul
③ Mrs. Nina's role -
  • Email Paul
  • Think about ideas for what direction to go in when we get back.
Contacts email Mrs. Nina calls - 2 per week

have little success. He may become turned off to therapy because it seems to him that therapy doesn't work. This could have unfortunate consequences in the future when the child (or adult) is finally ready to make changes. He may look back on his therapy experiences negatively. Recalling therapy as simply a time when he was "dragged" to speech by his parents even though he got nothing out of it will not encourage him to want to approach therapy again. As a result, he may be very reluctant to pursue treatment even if the time is finally right for him to make real and substantive progress. Therefore, we try to help parents and others learn that children will *always* have the opportunity to come to treatment when they are ready. It is never too late for children (or adults) to learn to improve their communication abilities — or their communication attitudes — through successful, effective therapy that addresses the entire stuttering disorder.

Open door policy

For children who are learning to manage their stuttering, it can be very comforting for them to stay in contact with a supportive and knowledgeable SLP, even if they are not presently enrolled in therapy. An "open door" approach to ongoing therapy allows for this feeling of security because it gives the child the option of meeting with you when needed rather than on an arbitrary schedule that is designed mainly to keep the child on the caseload. Fortunately, clincians in any work setting can provide this type of flexible service. Even in the schools, you can manage paperwork by offering periods of "monitoring" or "consultation" service delivery. We may also recommend a treatment schedule of just a few hours per month. This allows a child to take breaks from formal speech therapy without being discharged from your caseload. It also provides an opportunity for a child to return to direct services on a more regular schedule whenever he is ready.

Other options

Regardless of whether or not we recommend therapy for a child who stutters, many children who stutter—and their families—can benefit from forms of intervention other than formal speech treatment. As we will discuss in more detail toward the end of this book, we have worked with many children who have benefited from participating in self-help support organizations for people who stutter. Such support systems can help children who stutter truly realize that they are not the only one facing the challenges of stuttering; there are literally millions of other people who have experienced the same types of fears and frustrations they have experienced. The knowledge that they are not alone in their struggles can help children who stutter find the strength to confront their feelings about stuttering and persevere in treatment even when they feel that they are not making progress.

Support organizations can also help parents come to terms with their children's stuttering in a way that we often cannot (due to various factors such as the difficulty of maintaining contact with parents when we are working in the school setting). When parents of children who stutter can talk with other parents of children who stutter—or even when they can read personal stories written by other parents—they can begin to find hope for themselves and for their children. Therefore, we try to introduce all of the children we work with to support groups, either as an adjunct to therapy or, in cases where therapy is not possible or appropriate, as a substitute for therapy until the child is ready or willing to participate in treatment.

Deciding to Recommend Therapy

Although there are certainly times when the children we evaluate may not be ready for therapy, there are *many* other times when they are ready and willing to work to improve their speech fluency and communication skills. In fact, although we have reviewed a number of reasons that children may not be referred for treatment, we find that the majority of children we evaluate do indeed need therapy. Thus, more often than not, we make the recommendation that the child should be enrolled in therapy and we prepare a therapy plan that is tailored to the needs of each individual child.

How often should I see the child?

Because each child who stutters is different and requires individualized case decisions, it is impossible to make blanket recommendations about the number of times children who stutter should be seen in treatment per week or per month. Still, we can highlight a number of issues you can consider when making treatment recommendations for school-age children who stutter.

Two questions to ask yourself when deciding how often to see a child for therapy are: "How much therapy time can best meet the needs of this individual child?" and "What is the best service delivery model for this individual child?" You must be aware of *how* you will be providing therapy when making recommendations about therapy frequency and time. In private settings, one session per week may be enough if the child and family can be seen on an intensive one-to-one basis. You may also wish to include additional group sessions with other children who stutter when the child is ready for that type of peer interaction.

In school settings, however, more time is typically required. In the schools, you must carefully consider the service delivery model (or combination of models) that you think is best for each child. The amount of time needed for treatment will differ, depending upon whether you will be providing direct therapy in the classroom or seeing the child outside the classroom on a "pull out" basis. Similarly, the optimal session duration will depend upon whether the child is seen individually or in a group. If a group is going to be the best setting for the child, you must consider whether the group will consist entirely of children who stutter or whether there will be children with other types of speech and language disorders in the group. You must also consider whether classroom teachers, parents, and others will be available for consultation, planning, and collaboration. Finally, you must consider whether you plan to monitor the child's progress through direct contact or visits with school personnel so you can include this monitoring time in your treatment plan as necessary.

It is by considering all of these factors that you will be able to arrive at a treatment duration recommendation that will be most beneficial to the children you serve. Of course, because of the complexity and long-term nature of the disorder, we believe that children who stutter should never be given the "minimal" amount of therapy for which they are eligible. When in doubt, we feel it is best to err on the side of more therapy rather than less so children who stutter will have the time and opportunity to gain the maximal benefit from treatment.

What am I going to say at the parent conference?

Even though we have met with or spoken with a child's parents a number of times during the assessment process, the first "formal" meeting among parents, SLP, and others (depending upon the setting) can take on a great deal of importance. The child and his family may have to assimilate a lot of new information, including the fact that the child may not be likely to "outgrow" stuttering. Depending upon where a family is in their process of coming to terms with their child's stuttering, more than one meeting may be necessary. Sensitivity to the family's needs in the early stages of therapy will help to ensure that the family is "on board" with the goals and procedures of therapy.

During the initial meeting(s), you can review assessment procedures, test results, determination of eligibility (either for treatment in schools or for insurance coverage), treatment recommendations, and the overall goals to be addressed for both the child and family. This is a great deal of information, and it can be overwhelming for the parents and even for you. Because of this, we prefer not to give parents too much information in the initial meetings. The key question in our minds when we enter the diagnostic evaluation is whether or not the child needs treatment. Not surprisingly, this question is also foremost in the parents' minds. Therefore, we try to focus on this issue when we begin to meet with parents.

During the conference(s), you want to help the parents understand your recommendation for treatment and why you have made that recommendation. Some parents may want specific details supporting the recommendation, though others may not. Try to give the parents the level of detail they require for understanding this initial step in the process. An outline of a suggested initial parent conference can be found on page 116 (Appendix 3M). Additional, less formal meetings can then be arranged to educate parents about stuttering, to discuss the process and philosophy of therapy, and most importantly, to answer parents' questions and concerns after they have had a chance to consider your initial recommendations. A suggested outline of this feedback conference is on page 117 (Appendix 3N).

During the initial conference, you should try to *listen as much as you talk*. You have a lot of information to convey to parents about their child's speech skills, and about the disorder of stuttering itself. All of this information will not help parents, however, if they are not ready to hear it. It is essential to listen to parents and use counseling skills such as reflecting and validating their concerns so they can assimilate the information you provide. This will help them become active partners in the therapy process.

You may be the first person to listen to the parents and acknowledge their concerns about their child's stuttering. You must realize that up to this point, parents may not have had any support in facing their concerns about their child's speech. The pediatrician may have told them "he will outgrow it," well-meaning relatives may have given advice such as "just have him slow down," and others may have told them to just ignore the problem. Now you are asking them to face the stuttering, and, in many cases, to accept the fact that their child may not develop completely "normal" fluency. Not surprisingly, this can be difficult news for parents to hear, and you need to help them come to terms with what you have told them about their child's prognosis before you inundate them with facts and figures about the stuttering disorder. Thus, you need to approach the initial conference cautiously and slowly, keeping in mind that your overriding goal is to help them begin to understand the nature of their child's stuttering rather than to simply provide information about the stuttering disorder.

Treatment Coverage and Eligibility

Every clinical setting has specific rules governing the provision of speech therapy services for children with communication disorders, and you need to be familiar with these guidelines when making treatment recommendations. In this section, we discuss the impact of these rules for determining treatment eligibility in the public schools (based on IDEA) and the provision of insurance coverage for children being seen in the private sector.

Don't I need a severity rating to get the child qualified for treatment?

Many clinicians are accustomed to providing a severity rating, derived from a "standardized testing instrument," to demonstrate a child's need for treatment. Indeed, many states or districts have developed their own entry and exit criteria for treatment for communication disorders that rely on such ratings. According to the IDEA, however, this is not only unnecessary, but specifically not within the spirit of the law. For clinicians working in a state or district that does define a severity rating or set stuttering frequency as a primary factor for determining eligibility for speech therapy, it is important to note that this practice is not consistent with the intent of IDEA '97.

In actuality, IDEA requires *multiple* forms of assessment from a variety of sources. These sources may include standardized tests, of course,

Schools Alert: "Eligibility, Schmeligibility"

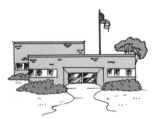

One of the most common concerns we hear from school-based clinicians working with children who stutter is that they cannot qualify children for treatment even though they know the children need that treatment. For example, we are told that a child "did not stutter enough" during the evaluation to meet the district's guidelines. Or, we hear that a child is a "straight-A" student "who must not be experiencing any educational difficulties and, therefore, does not qualify for treatment" even though he stutters severely and experiences many negative consequences as a result of his stuttering. Although these situations seem to occur frequently, they are not consistent with current regulations regarding the eligibility of children who stutter for treatment. More importantly, these situations do not provide sufficient justification for a child to be denied treatment if the clinician can document the need for that treatment.

The legislation that allows us to qualify children for treatment based on their need for intervention rather than their grades or frequency of stuttering is the Individuals with Disabilities Education Act (IDEA), Part B regulations of 1997. Many school clinicians are familiar with the phrase "adversely affects educational performance" as the key criterion dictating when children can receive special education services such as speech therapy. Oddly, though the phrase is widely recognized, it is poorly understood. It has never truly been defined in federal regulations, and this has opened up the opportunity for clinicians (and administrators) to interpret the phrase in different ways.

Some have interpreted this key phrase to mean that IDEA requires that stuttering must adversely affect a child's academics (interpreted as grades) in order for him to be eligible for treatment. Nothing could be further from the truth. The 1997 reauthorization of IDEA actually increased the accessibility of services for children who stutter by emphasizing the need to view speech disorders not just in terms of their impact on a child's grades and classroom performance, but also in terms of their impact on other aspects of a child's life. Specifically, the Department of Education stated in 1990 that "a child's educational performance should include nonacademic as well as academic areas." This means that a child who stutters cannot be denied services simply because he or she is achieving passing grades in academic classes. The determination of eligibility should be based on factors beyond the observable characteristics of speech.

but they are not limited to them. In fact, the IDEA legislation reviews several limitations to norm-referenced tests as the determining factors for eligibility for services and encourages clinicians to use interviews with the child, targeted observations, information from parents and teachers of a child (including adaptive behavior checklists), samples of a child's classroom work or participation, and any information gathered that is pertinent to the child's progress in the general curriculum. In other words, the IDEA supports the notion of portfolio-based assessment such as that described earlier in this chapter.

What happens if the child is not eligible through traditional assessment procedures?

When a child appears ineligible for treatment following traditional assessment procedures, the assessment team has an option of also utilizing "professional judgment." (According to IDEA, the assessment team includes, but is not limited to, the child's parents, at least one regular education teacher, at least one special education teacher, an individual who can interpret evaluation results, and if appropriate, the child). The use of "professional judgment" allows the team to determine that a child is eligible for treatment even in the absence of traditional measures of deficits in the child's speech fluency. Thus, if a child is experiencing difficulty interacting with other children, or if he does not participate fully in class, or if he exhibits negative affective and cognitive reactions to stuttering, then he can be deemed eligible for treatment even if he does not demonstrate severe stuttering on a standardized instrument. As long as the assessment team can document through formal or informal procedures that the child needs therapy, then it is appropriate—and consistent with current legislation—for the team to recommend therapy.

What about three-year re-evaluations?

Three-year re-evaluations are a part of the procedures clinicians must follow when working in the public schools. Sometimes, clinicians tell us that they are concerned a child may not (re)qualify for treatment at his three-year evaluation specifically because of the progress he is making in therapy. In other words, clinicians may fear that the child will no longer meet arbitrary eligibility criteria because his communication skills have improved, even if he is not ready to be dismissed from treatment, and even if more work remains to be done. Fortunately, given what we now know about the IDEA legislation, we can say that triennial assessments provide an excellent opportunity to document the changes the child has achieved without worrying about whether he will be disqualified from further therapy.

What if stuttering isn't covered by insurance?

Stuttering is often included in the list of exclusions for many major insurance programs. The reasons for this are not clear, though there are several possible explanations. First, denial of insurance coverage may be related to the fact that stuttering often starts (and sometimes stops) in early childhood. This has caused most insurers to consider stuttering a "developmental" disorder. Although the term itself is not particularly enlightening, it does provide the justification the insurance company needs for denying coverage. The difficulties with insurance coverage for stuttering may also be related to the fact that mandated speech therapy services for stuttering are provided in the schools. As a result, insurance companies may determine that they do not need to pay for the services since families have access to therapy through the school system. Finally, another common reason for insurance denial is the idea that stuttering treatment is not "medically necessary." Technically of course, this is true. Stuttering is not a life-threatening condition, though it can have serious consequences for people who stutter and their families. Nevertheless, it is the job of insurance companies to keep their own costs down and denying or restricting coverage for a disorder such as stuttering may be one way in which they seek to do this.

Although there are no guarantees about obtaining insurance coverage for stuttering, we have found it helpful to educate parents about their rights in applying for insurance coverage, including the appeals process. Generally, tenacious families who appeal insurance denials are more likely to get at least partial payment for therapy than families who simply accept their insurance company's denial without appealing. Often, clinicians and pediatricians can write letters of support explaining the need for therapy and emphasizing the true impact of the disorder on the child's ability to communicate, to interact with others, to succeed in school, and to achieve better quality of life. Of course, these letters are not always successful, and the insurance company may only authorize a limited number or duration of sessions. Still, the effort can help to educate the insurance company's review panel about stuttering and may increase the likelihood of coverage. And, for many families, obtaining coverage for even a few sessions may make a significant difference in their abilities to enroll their children in treatment.

Private Sector Alert: Who's Going to Pay for This?

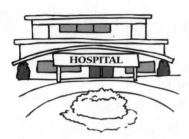

While clinicians working in the public school system may need to focus on eligibility criteria and current legislation such as IDEA to determine whether a child can receive treatment, clinicians working in the private sector have a different set of concerns. Speech therapy provided in the private sector is not free, and clinicians must constantly be aware of the costs of their services for families of children who stutter. Because stuttering therapy is often an open-ended experience with no easily definable duration, it can be difficult for families to commit the financial resources necessary to enroll a child in therapy or to maintain therapy over the long term. In some cases, families may have access to medical insurance that will cover the costs of treatment; however, insurance coverage is far from certain. Even in cases where coverage can be obtained, there are often limits to the number or duration of sessions that are provided. The challenges of obtaining coverage for treatment are faced every day by clinicians in the private sector, and there are no easy answers.

Fortunately, organizations such as ASHA, the Stuttering Foundation of America (SFA), and the National Stuttering Association (NSA) have prepared brochures and handouts designed to help families obtain coverage for their child's treatment. These organizations, as well as other helpful resources, are listed in Appendix 2A, pages 45 and 46.

What if the family can't afford treatment?

In the end, there will be some families who simply cannot afford to enroll their children in private therapy. Of course, in such cases, families will always have access to treatment through the public schools; however, there may be reasons that a child may not wish to participate in therapy at school (e.g., unwillingness to be taken out of class, lack of access to a clinician with expertise in stuttering, scheduling difficulties). If the child cannot receive school-based or private-sector treatment, then it is important for you to help parents understand that all is not lost.

As we mentioned earlier, we take a long-term view of the stuttering disorder. Because managing stuttering is a lifelong process, we know that children who stutter can learn to improve their communication abilities at any time in the future. Thus, even if a child cannot participate in treatment at a particular point in his development, he will still have many other opportunities in his life to address his speech difficulties.

This is also a situation where we find it useful to draw upon other resources. Specifically, you can connect families (all families—not just those who have difficulty paying for treatment) with support organizations such as the National Stuttering Association and the Stuttering Foundation of America. As we mentioned before, such organizations can help parents and their children learn more about stuttering, and the support people who stutter receive through these groups can help them learn to deal with their stuttering in a positive and proactive manner. In this way, you can provide a meaningful service to people who stutter even if you cannot treat them directly. We say more about the valuable role of support systems in Chapter 7.

Summary

In this chapter, we have attempted to review the goals and procedures for evaluating children who stutter and making recommendations for treatment in different clinical settings. We approached this process by asking questions about where the child came from, where he has been, where he is now, and where he is going. The information we collect through the evaluation is based on a variety of methods, including standardized testing, formal and informal observation, portfolio assessment, and interviews with individuals who are important in the child's life. Ultimately, we seek to answer the question of whether the child should be enrolled in treatment by trying to determine an appropriate set of goals for helping the child improve his speech fluency, attitudes, and communication skills. In the next chapters, we will review the specific treatment procedures we use to achieve these goals.

Stuttering Case History

Personal Information

Child

Name _____   Check one: Male _____   Female _____

Date of Birth _____   Age _____   Grade _____

Home Address _____   Home Phone _____

City, State, Zip _____   Referred by _____

Parent(s)/Guardian(s)

Mother _____ Occupation _____ Day Phone _____

Father _____ Occupation _____ Day Phone _____

Other People in the Household

Name _____   Age _____   Relationship _____

Name _____   Age _____   Relationship _____

Name _____   Age _____   Relationship _____

Name _____   Age _____   Relationship _____

History of Speech/Language Problems

1. Please describe your child's speaking difficulty in your own words. _____

   _____

2. At what age was this problem first noticed? _____

3. Who first noticed the problem? _____

4. How has the problem changed since that time? _____

   _____

5. Do you have difficulty understanding your child?   Yes   No

6. Do other people have difficulty understanding your child?   Yes   No

7. Has your child previously been assessed for speech/language concerns?   Yes   No

   If *yes*, please describe. _____

   _____

8. Has your child received any prior speech/language therapy?   Yes   No

   If *yes*, where? _____   By whom? _____

   For how long? _____   Focus of Treatment _____

   Results of Treatment _____

   _____

9. Have any other family members had speech/language problems?   Yes   No

   Please indicate the person's relationship to your child and the nature of the problem.

   _____

   _____

Medical History and Current Health Status

1. Was there anything remarkable about the mother's health during
   pregnancy or delivery?   Yes   No

   If *yes*, please describe. _____

2. Was there anything remarkable about your child's condition at birth?   Yes   No

   If *yes*, please describe. _____

3. Does your child have developmental concerns other than speech/language?   Yes   No

   If *yes*, please describe. _____

4. At approximately what age did your child begin to:

   walk _____   use words _____   combine words _____

5. Has your child experienced ear infections?   Yes   No

   If *yes*, approximately how often? (Circle one.) Rarely   Occasionally   Frequently

   Do you feel that your child hears normally? Yes   No

   Explain. _____

   Has your child's hearing ever been tested? Yes   No

   Results _____   Date _____

6. Please indicate if your child has experienced the following medical problems.

Chicken Pox _____	Tonsilitis _____	Vision Problems _____
Pneumonia _____	Headaches _____	High Fever _____
Seizures _____	Allergies _____	Asthma _____

7. Describe any illnesses, accidents, injuries, or hospitalizations (include age and treatment).

_____

_____

_____

8. How often do the following behaviors occur?   (O = Often, S = Sometimes, N = Never)

a.	inattentiveness	O	S	N	g. frustration	O	S	N
b.	hyperactivity	O	S	N	h. strong fears	O	S	N
c.	nervousness	O	S	N	i. excessive neatness	O	S	N
d.	sensitivity	O	S	N	j. excessive shyness	O	S	N
e.	perfectionism	O	S	N	k. lack of confidence	O	S	N
f.	excitability	O	S	N	l. competitiveness	O	S	N

9. What is your child's current health?   good _____   fair _____   poor _____

10. Is your child currently taking any medications?   Yes   No   If *yes*, please list.

_____

11. Does your child have any other medical diagnoses or concerns? _____

_____

Speech Fluency and Stuttering

1. When did your child first start stuttering? (Please be as specific as possible.)

_____

2. What did the stuttering sound like when it first began?_____

_____

3. Describe how your child's speech sounds now. _____

_____

4. What seems to help your child when he or she is stuttering? _____

_____

5. Has your child ever demonstrated any:

   awareness of stuttering   _____   physical tension during stuttering _____

   frustration about speaking _____   complaints that he/she "can't talk" _____

   Please describe. _____

_____

6. Has your child ever been teased about stuttering?   Yes   No

    If *yes*, please describe. _____

    _____

7. Has your child ever discussed his/her speaking difficulties with you?   Yes   No

    If *yes*, please describe. _____

    _____

8. Does anyone in your child's immediate family stutter?   Yes   No

    If *yes*, please name. _____

    Anyone on child's mother's side? _____   Anyone on child's father's side? _____

    Please describe the relative(s) stuttering. _____

    _____

9. Have you or your child ever known another person who stutters?   Yes   No

    If *yes*, who? _____

10. How does your child's stuttering affect his/her:

    academic performance? _____

    participation in school activities? _____

    interaction with other children? _____

    interaction with family members? _____

    willingness to talk and communicate? _____

    self-esteem or attitude toward self? _____

11. What else do you think we should know about your child (e.g., hobbies, interests, social skills)?

    _____

    _____

    _____

Example Stuttering Case History

Personal Information

Child

Name _____Thomas_____   Check one: Male __X__ Female ____

Date of Birth _____   Age __7__ Grade __1__

Home Address _____   Home Phone _____

City, State, Zip _____   Referred by ___speech teacher___

Parent(s)/Guardian(s)

Mother ___Suzanne___ Occupation ___Sales___ Day Phone _____

Father ___Joseph___ Occupation _Superintendant_ Day Phone _____

Other People in the Household

Name ___Adrianne___ Age __4__ Relationship ___sister___

Name ___Scotty___ Age __9__ Relationship ___brother___

Name _____ Age ____ Relationship _____

Name _____ Age ____ Relationship _____

History of Speech/Language Problems

1. Please describe your child's speaking difficulty in your own words. _Thomas repeats sounds at the start of many of his sentences._

2. At what age was this problem first noticed? _about 4 or so_

3. Who first noticed the problem? _I did (Mom)_

4. How has the problem changed since that time? _It used to come and go. Now it's always present._

5. Do you have difficulty understanding your child?   Yes   (No)

6. Do other people have difficulty understanding your child?   Yes   (No)

7. Has your child previously been assessed for speech/language concerns? (Yes)   No

   If *yes*, please describe. _In preschool, he had some trouble with his beginning and ending sounds._

8. Has your child received any prior speech/language therapy?   (Yes)   No

   If *yes*, where? ____private therapy____   By whom? _____

   For how long? _____6 mos._____   Focus of Treatment ____sounds____

   Results of Treatment ____Thomas can be understood all the time now.____

   _____

9. Have any other family members had speech/language problems?   (Yes)   No

   Please indicate the person's relationship to your child and the nature of the problem.

   _____Dad had speech when he was young for his sounds._____

   _____

Medical History and Current Health Status

1. Was there anything remarkable about the mother's health during
   pregnancy or delivery?   Yes   (No)

   If *yes*, please describe. _____

2. Was there anything remarkable about your child's condition at birth?   Yes   (No)

   If *yes*, please describe. _____

3. Does your child have developmental concerns other than speech/language?   Yes   (No)

   If *yes*, please describe. _____

4. At approximately what age did your child begin to:

   walk <u>1 year</u>   use words <u>1 year</u>   combine words <u>18 mos.</u>

5. Has your child experienced ear infections?   Yes   (No)

   If *yes*, approximately how often? (Circle one.)   Rarely   Occasionally   Frequently

   Do you feel that your child hears normally? (Yes)   No

   Explain. _____

   Has your child's hearing ever been tested?   (Yes)   No

   Results _____normal_____   Date _____

6. Please indicate if your child has experienced the following medical problems.

Chicken Pox	_____	Tonsilitis	_____	Vision Problems	_____
Pneumonia	_____	Headaches	_____	High Fever	_____
Seizures	_____	Allergies	__X__	Asthma	_____

7. Describe any illnesses, accidents, injuries, or hospitalizations (include age and treatment).

   _____ broken arm, age 6 _____

   _____

   _____

8. How often do the following behaviors occur?   (O = Often, S = Sometimes, N = Never)

a.	inattentiveness	O	(S)	N	g.	frustration	O S (N)
b.	hyperactivity	O	S	(N)	h.	strong fears	O S (N)
c.	nervousness	O	(S)	(N)	i.	excessive neatness	O (S) (N)
d.	sensitivity	O	(S)	N	j.	excessive shyness	O (S) N
e.	perfectionism	O	(S)	N	k.	lack of confidence	O (S) N
f.	excitability	O	(S)	N	l.	competitiveness	(O) S N

9. What is your child's current health?   good __X__   fair _____   poor _____

10. Is your child currently taking any medications?   (Yes)   No   If *yes*, please list.

    _____ allergy med as needed _____

11. Does your child have any other medical diagnoses or concerns? _____ No _____

Speech Fluency and Stuttering

1. When did your child first start stuttering? (Please be as specific as possible.)

   _____ When he was 4 and we were on vacation. _____

2. What did the stuttering sound like when it first began?___ Thomas had trouble _____

   _____ getting the words out. _____

3. Describe how your child's speech sounds now. _____ More repetitions _____

   _____

4. What seems to help your child when he or she is stuttering? _____ I don't know. ___

   _____

5. Has your child ever demonstrated any:

   awareness of stuttering   ___X___   physical tension during stuttering _____

   frustration about speaking _____   complaints that he/she "can't talk" _____

   Please describe. _____ Covers his mouth, whispers sometimes. _____

   _____

6. Has your child ever been teased about stuttering?   Yes   (No)

If *yes*, please describe. ___Not that I know of but his cousin asked him why he "talked like that"___

7. Has your child ever discussed his/her speaking difficulties with you?   Yes   (No)

If *yes*, please describe. _____

8. Does anyone in your child's immediate family stutter?   Yes   (No)

If *yes*, please name. _____

Anyone on child's mother's side? ___Yes___   Anyone on child's father's side? _____

Please describe the relative(s) stuttering. ___Thomas' great aunt. She seems to get stuck on her words.___

9. Have you or your child ever known another person who stutters?   Yes   (No)

If *yes*, who? _____

10. How does your child's stuttering affect his/her:

     academic performance? ___No___

     participation in school activities? ___not sure___

     interaction with other children? ___He's shy sometimes.___

     interaction with family members? ___No___

     willingness to talk and communicate? ___No___

     self-esteem or attitude toward self? ___not sure___

11. What else do you think we should know about your child (e.g., hobbies, interests, social skills)?

___He likes action figures. He is loving and playful with his siblings. He has a great sense of humor.___

Parent Perceptions ————————————————————

This form is designed to gather information about your perceptions of your child's stuttering (and past therapy if applicable). It should be completed separately by each parent.

Child's Name _____ **Age** _____ **Grade** _____

Person Completing Form _____ **Date** _____

Relationship to child _____

I have heard that stuttering is caused by _____

_____

It is my belief that stuttering is caused by _____

_____

Some questions I have about stuttering are _____

_____

_____

My child shows awareness of his/her speech difficulties.   Yes   No

If *yes*, please describe what your child has said or done to make you think he/she is aware?

_____

_____

I notice that my child has the most difficulty talking when _____

_____

_____

When my child stutters, other people react by _____

_____

_____

I feel _____ when I watch my child struggling with speech, and I want _____

_____

_____

When my child stutters, I try to help by _____

_____

I think the goal of stuttering therapy should be _____

_____

Parent Perceptions, continued ───────────────

My child's teachers have knowledge about stuttering.   Yes   No   I don't know

My child's teachers have tried to help by _____

_____

The most important thing for someone to know about my child is _____

_____

I think my child is ready to be in speech therapy.   Yes   No

If *no*, please explain. _____

I feel at this time that my child's level of motivation for working on his/her speech is _____

_____

_____

I think I can best help my child by _____

_____

As a parent of a child who stutters, what I want most right now is _____

_____

My wish for my child in five years is _____

_____

Please answer the following questions if your child has received therapy in the past.

The two most important things I learned from my child's other speech therapists were

_____

_____

In my child's past therapy, he/she worked on _____

_____

The most helpful aspect of my child's past therapy was _____

_____

The least helpful aspect of my child's past therapy was _____

_____

I am satisfied with the level of effort my child has put into speech therapy.   Yes   No

Example Parent Perceptions

This form is designed to gather information about your perceptions of your child's stuttering (and past therapy if applicable). It should be completed separately by each parent.

Child's Name _____Thomas_____   **Age** _7_   **Grade** _1_

Person Completing Form _____Suzanne_____   **Date** _____

Relationship to child _____mother_____

I have heard that stuttering is caused by _____parents talking too fast._____

It is my belief that stuttering is caused by _____talking faster than you can think._____

Some questions I have about stuttering are _____What can I do to help my child speak more fluently?_____

My child shows awareness of his/her speech difficulties.   (Yes)   No

If *yes*, please describe what your child has said or done to make you think he/she is aware?
_____He covers his mouth sometimes._____
_____Sometimes it seems like he says fewer words when he is repeating a lot._____

I notice that my child has the most difficulty talking when _____he is excited, tired, or fighting for attention._____

When my child stutters, other people react by _____Sometimes talking slower to him._____
_____Most of the time, there aren't many reactions._____

I feel _____helpless_____ when I watch my child struggling with speech, and I want _____to know how we can help him._____

When my child stutters, I try to help by _____making eye contact and letting him finish._____

I think the goal of stuttering therapy should be _____managing his speaking to near-normal most of the time._____

My child's teachers have knowledge about stuttering. (Yes) & (No)   I don't know

My child's teachers have tried to help by __giving him time to talk.__

_____

The most important thing for someone to know about my child is _____

_____ __He is fun-loving and usually happy.__ _____

I think my child is ready to be in speech therapy.   (Yes)   No

If *no*, please explain. __I think he wonders about his speech.__

I feel at this time that my child's level of motivation for working on his/her speech is _____

_____ __I really don't know.__ _____

_____

I think I can best help my child by __getting him help and being patient while he__

_____ __goes through this.__ _____

As a parent of a child who stutters, what I want most right now is _____

_____ __that he will outgrow this so he won't retreat socially.__

My wish for my child in five years is __that he will be able to say what he wants to__

_____ __say, that he will have friends, and that he will be happy.__

Please answer the following questions if your child has received therapy in the past.

The two most important things I learned from my child's other speech therapists were

__In preschool, when he was having some trouble during his "sounds" therapy,__

__the clinician told us to be "slow & easy" with our speech.__

In my child's past therapy, he/she worked on __sounds only.__

_____

The most helpful aspect of my child's past therapy was __having someone to talk to.__

_____

The least helpful aspect of my child's past therapy was _____

_____ __we never addressed the stuttering.__

I am satisfied with the level of effort my child has put into speech therapy. (Yes)   No

Previous Therapy History ————————————————————

If you have ever had speech therapy to help you with your stuttering, this form is for you! You get to tell about what you liked and didn't like, what you learned, and didn't learn.

Name _____   **Date** _____

Age _____   **Grade** _____

The last time I went to speech therapy was _____

_____

The main reason I went to speech therapy was _____

_____

We worked on _____

_____

The two most important things I learned from my other speech teacher(s) were _____

_____

_____

The two most important things *my parents* learned from my other speech teacher(s) were

_____

_____

The best thing about my past therapy was _____

_____

The worst thing about my past therapy was _____

_____

My other speech teacher(s) gave me practice assignments to do at home.   Yes   No

When they gave me homework, I did it: (Circle one)

     not at all   a little   some   a lot

I believe that speech therapy can help my talking: (Circle one)

     not at all   a little   some   a lot

I do/do not (circle one) think therapy can help me because _____

_____

I think I stutter because _____

_____

One question I have about stuttering is _____

_____

Some things I do now that help my speech are _____

_____

_____

Something I want from therapy now is _____

_____

_____

Example Previous Therapy History

If you have ever had speech therapy to help you with your stuttering, this form is for you! You get to tell about what you liked and didn't like, what you learned, and didn't learn.

Name _____Carrie_____   **Date** _____

Age ___10___   **Grade** ___5___

The last time I went to speech therapy was _____last year._____

The main reason I went to speech therapy was _____my mom kept signing me up._____

We worked on _____easy speech, relaxing._____

The two most important things I learned from my other speech teacher(s) were _____

_____how to go easy on my words_____

_____not to push harder when I get stuck_____

The two most important things *my parents* learned from my other speech teacher(s) were

_____not to make me use my tools_____

_____not to get crazy about my speech_____

The best thing about my past therapy was _____sometimes we had pizza and treats._____

The worst thing about my past therapy was _____we were reading out loud all the time._____

My other speech teacher(s) gave me practice assignments to do at home.   (Yes)   No

When they gave me homework, I did it: (Circle one)

       not at all   (a little)   some   a lot

I believe that speech therapy can help my talking: (Circle one)

       not at all   a little   (some)   a lot

I (do) do not (circle one) think therapy can help me because I really want it to.
_____

I think I stutter because   I have no clue. Maybe because I talk fast sometimes.
_____

One question I have about stuttering is   Why me? Will it ever go away?
_____

Some things I do now that help my speech are easy beginnings and taking my time.
_____
_____

Something I want from therapy now is   What should I do when I get really stuck?
_____
_____

Speech Disfluency Count Sheet

Name _____

Birthdate _____ Eval. Date _____ Age _____ Clinician _____

Overall Disfl. Frequency/Severity Rating _____

Stuttered Disfl. % / Types _____ Nonstutt. Disfl. % / Types _____

Situation: _____

Syllables/Words (circle one)

Type	#
I	
Rv	
Rp	
Rw	
Rs	
P	
B	
O	
%	

Situation: _____

Syllables/Words (circle one)

Type	#
I	
Rv	
Rp	
Rw	
Rs	
P	
B	
O	
%	

Situation: _____

Syllables/Words (circle one)

Type	#
I	
Rv	
Rp	
Rw	
Rs	
P	
B	
O	
%	

Situation: _____

Syllables/Words (circle one)

Type	#
I	
Rv	
Rp	
Rw	
Rs	
P	
B	
O	
%	

Nonstutt. Disfl.	Stuttered Disfl.
I Interjection	Rw Word rep.
Rv Revision	Rs Sound/syllable rep.
Rp Phrase Rep.	P Prolongation
O Other (specify)	B Block

Copyright © 2003 LinguiSystems, Inc.

Notes _____

Appendix 3G
The Source for School Age Stuttering

Example Speech Disfluency Count Sheet

Name Sample School-age Child Age 9 yrs., 5 mos.

Birthdate _____ Eval. Date _____ Clinician _____

Overall Disfl. Frequency/Severity Rating Conv: Mild, Reading/Story: Severe

Stuttered Disfl. % / Types Rs and P   Nonstutt. Disfl. % / Types 1 in story

---

Situation: Conversation with Father — Syllables/**Words** (circle one)

Type	#
I	2
Rv	0
Rp	0
Rw	0
Rs	4
P	4
B	0
O	0
%	2 / 8

10% total

Situation: Conversation with Peer — Syllables/**Words** (circle one)

Type	#
I	0
Rv	0
Rp	2
Rw	0
Rs	3
P	6
B	1
O	0
%	2 / 10

12% total

Situation: Reading (Three Bears) — Syllables/**Words** (circle one)

Type	#
I	2
Rv	0
Rp	0
Rw	0
Rs	12
P	11
B	0
O	0
%	2 / 23

25% total

Situation: Story Retell (Three Bears) — Syllables/**Words** (circle one)

Type	#
I	11
Rv	0
Rp	1
Rw	0
Rs	12
P	8
B	0
O	0
%	12 / 20

32% total

Nonstutt. Disfl.	Stuttered Disfl.
I Interjection	Rw Word rep.
Rv Revision	Rs Sound/syllable rep.
Rp Phrase Rep.	P Prolongation
O Other (specify)	B Block

Copyright © 2003 LinguiSystems, Inc.

Notes Very fast speaking rate for both child and father; prolongation approx. 1/2 to 1 second long. Minimal tension evident during disfluencies when in conversation with father or with peer. Considerably more tension and struggle during reading and story retell situations; duration 1 - 1 1/2 seconds. Frequent eye blinks evident discomfort during story retell (possible language issue?).

Appendix 3H
The Source for School-Age Stuttering

Teacher Checklist—Stuttering

Some students stutter or hesitate when they speak. This may interfere with communication both in and out of the classroom. This type of speech problem warrants further evaluation. Please help me gain a better overall view of this student's speech skills by completing the following information and returning to me by _____.
Thank you!

Speech-Language Pathologist _____   **Phone/Room** _____

Student _____   Birthdate _____   Age _____   Grade _____

School _____   Teacher _____   Section _____   Date _____

Follow-up is important, so I would like to observe this child in several different situations. Please list when this student:

Goes to lunch _____   Shares in the classroom _____

Attends gym class _____   Interacts with peers   _____

Please let me know the best way to contact you: Days/Times _____

E-mail _____   Phone _____

General Information

1. Compared to his/her peers, this student: (Check all that apply.)

   _____ doesn't mind talking in class

   _____ tries to avoid speaking in class. (does not speak if called upon; asks few questions.)

   _____ speaks with little or no outward signs of frustration or embarrassment

   _____ sometimes uses gestures to avoid speaking

   _____ is difficult to understand in class

   _____ demonstrates frustration when speaking (Please describe.) _____

   _____ exhibits academic performance at an average or above-average level

2. This student is disfluent or stutters when he/she: (Check all that apply.)

   _____ begins the first word of a sentence   _____ speaks to the class

   _____ speaks during an entire sentence   _____ gets upset

   _____ uses little words   _____ shares ideas or tells a story

   _____ uses main words   _____ answers questions

   _____ talks with peers   _____ carries on a conversation

   _____ talks to adults   _____ reads aloud

   _____ other _____

3. Check any of the following behaviors you have noticed in this child's speech:

   _____ revisions (starting and stopping and starting over again)

   _____ frequent interjections (*um, like, you know*)

   _____ word repetitions (*we-we-we*)

   _____ phrase repetitions (*and then, and then*)

   _____ part-word repetitions (*ta-ta-take*)

   _____ prolongations (*nnnnobody*)

   _____ blocks (vocal tension/no speech comes out)

   _____ unusual face or body movments (visible tension, head nods, eye movements)

   _____ abnormal breathing patterns

   _____ other _____

In the Classroom

1. I do/do not (circle one) have concerns about this child's speech because _____

   _____

2. I observe the most disfluency when _____

3. When this child has difficulty speaking, he/she reacts by _____

   _____

4. When this child has difficulty speaking, I respond by _____

   _____

Perceptions About Stuttering

1. I have had prior experience with a child who stutters.   Yes   No

2. I feel that stuttering is caused by _____

3. Some questions I have about stuttering are _____

   _____

4. Some questions I have about how to help this child communicate effectively in the classroom

   include _____

   _____

5. I think the goal of stuttering therapy should be _____

6. The amount of knowledge I currently have regarding the disorder of stuttering is:

   nothing ⟵——————————————⟶ a lot
     1   2   3   4   5   6   7

7. My confidence level regarding dealing with stuttering in the classroom would be:

   not confident ⟵——————————————⟶ very confident
     1   2   3   4   5   6   7

8. My confidence level in identifying stuttering in children who stutter is:

   not confident ⟵——————————————⟶ very confident
     1   2   3   4   5   6   7

9. My confidence level in identifying avoidance behaviors in children who stutter is:

   not confident ⟵——————————————⟶ very confident
     1   2   3   4   5   6   7

10. My comfort level when communicating with this child is:

    Uncomfortable ⟵——————————————⟶ very comfortable
      1   2   3   4   5   6   7

Teacher Checklist—Stuttering, continued

Observations about this child

With Peers

1. How does this student relate with other students the same age? _____

   _____

2. Is this student teased or mimicked because of his/her speech?   Yes   No

   If *yes*, please describe. _____

3. When this child has difficulty speaking, the other children react by _____

   _____

4. Following a comment or teasing by a peer, how does this child react? _____

   _____

In General

1. Have other students or this students' parent(s) ever mentioned his/her fluency problems?   Yes   No

   If *yes*, what was discussed? _____

   _____

2. Has this student ever talked to you about his/her speech problem?   Yes   No

   If *yes*, what was discussed? _____

   _____

3. What other information might be helpful in looking at this student's fluency skills? _____

   _____

   _____

4. Do you have any other concerns regarding this child's speech and language, academic, or social skills?

   _____

   _____

Example Teacher Checklist—Stuttering

Some students stutter or hesitate when they speak. This may interfere with communication both in and out of the classroom. This type of speech problem warrants further evaluation. Please help me gain a better overall view of this student's speech skills by completing the following information and returning to me by _____.
Thank you!

Speech-Language Pathologist _____   **Phone/Room** _____

Student _Amanda_	**Birthdate** _____	**Age** _8.5_	**Grade** _3B_
School _____	**Teacher** _____	**Section** ____	**Date** ____

Follow-up is important, so I would like to observe this child in several different situations. Please list when this student:

Goes to lunch _11:50_	Shares in the classroom _10:15 Social Studies_
Attends gym class _2:40_	Interacts with peers _____

Please let me know the best way to contact you: Days/Times _____

          E-mail _____   Phone _____

General Information

1. Compared to his/her peers, this student: (Check all that apply.)
   - _____ doesn't mind talking in class
   - ✓ tries to avoid speaking in class. (does not speak if called upon; asks few questions.)
   - _____ speaks with little or no outward signs of frustration or embarrassment
   - _____ sometimes uses gestures to avoid speaking
   - ✓ is difficult to understand in class
   - ✓ demonstrates frustration when speaking (Please describe.) _Says "never mind"_
   - _____ exhibits academic performance at an average or above-average level

2. This student is disfluent or stutters when he/she: (Check all that apply.)

_____ begins the first word of a sentence	✓ speaks to the class
✓ speaks during an entire sentence	_____ gets upset
_____ uses little words	_____ shares ideas or tells a story
✓ uses main words	✓ answers questions
_____ talks with peers	_____ carries on a conversation
_____ talks to adults	_____ reads aloud
_____ other _____	

3. Check any of the following behaviors you have noticed in this child's speech:
   - _____ revisions (starting and stopping and starting over again)
   - ✓ frequent interjections (*um, like, you know*)
   - ✓ word repetitions (*we-we-we*)
   - _____ phrase repetitions (*and then, and then*)
   - ✓ part-word repetitions (*ta-ta-take*)
   - ✓ prolongations (*nnnnobody*)
   - ✓ blocks (vocal tension/no speech comes out)
   - ✓ unusual face or body movments (visible tension, head nods, eye movements)
   - ✓ abnormal breathing patterns
   - _____ other _____

In the Classroom

1. I do / do not (circle one) have concerns about this child's speech because _____
   she seems to be withdrawing.

2. I observe the most disfluency when _*she has a lot to say.*_

3. When this child has difficulty speaking, he/she reacts by _*being OK at first, but shutting down if it is really tough.*_

4. When this child has difficulty speaking, I respond by _*waiting for a while and then moving on so she doesn't have to continue struggling or get embarrassed.*_

Perceptions About Stuttering

1. I have had prior experience with a child who stutters. (Yes) No *but not this severe*

2. I feel that stuttering is caused by _*? Don't really know, but I think it's mostly emotional*_

3. Some questions I have about stuttering are _*Why does she have "good" days and "bad" days? How can I help?*_

4. Some questions I have about how to help this child communicate effectively in the classroom include _*What do I do when she is really stuck for a long time?*_

5. I think the goal of stuttering therapy should be _*to help children speak more fluently.*_

6. The amount of knowledge I currently have regarding the disorder of stuttering is:

   nothing ← ② → ③   4   5   6   7   a lot

   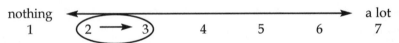

7. My confidence level regarding dealing with stuttering in the classroom would be:

   not confident ← ② → ③   4   5   6   7   very confident

   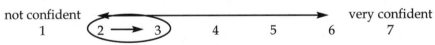

8. My confidence level in identifying stuttering in children who stutter is:

   not confident ← ②   3   4   5   6   7   very confident

   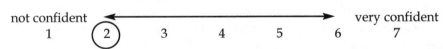

9. My confidence level in identifying avoidance behaviors in children who stutter is:

   not confident ← ②   3   4   5   6   7   very confident

   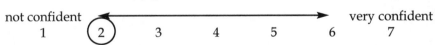

10. My comfort level when communicating with this child is:

    Uncomfortable ← 2   ③   4   5   6   7   very comfortable

    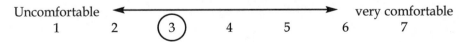

Observations about this child

With Peers

1. How does this student relate with other students the same age? *Does OK with most kids*
    _____

2. Is this student teased or mimicked because of his/her speech?   Yes   No

    If yes, please describe. *Not in class, but Mom reports the bus ride is bad.*

3. When this child has difficulty speaking, the other children react by _____
    _____ *some "staring" — but mostly waiting.* _____

4. Following a comment or teasing by a peer, how does this child react? *Seems embarrassed*
    _____

In General

1. Have other students or this students' parent(s) ever mentioned his/her fluency problems?   Yes   No

    If yes, what was discussed? *Parents discussed teasing with me recently.*
    _____

2. Has this student ever talked to you about his/her speech problem?   Yes   (No)

    If yes, what was discussed? _____
    _____

3. What other information might be helpful in looking at this student's fluency skills? _____
    _____ *She taps her foot a lot when reading. . . What is that about?* _____
    _____

4. Do you have any other concerns regarding this child's speech and language, academic, or social skills?
    _____ *We have lots of current-event oral presentations in second semester.*
    _____

My Thoughts About School

Name _____ **Grade** _____ **Age** _____ **Date** _____

Finish the sentences below.

When I am talking in class, the other kids usually _____

The hardest time for me to talk in school is _____

In school, some people that are hard to talk to are _____

In school, the easiest people to talk to are _____

When someone is trying to help me with my speech, they usually say/do_____

_____

When I have to talk in class, I usually _____

When I have trouble talking in class, the teacher usually _____

When I have trouble talking in school, my friends usually_____

When I have to give a presentation in class, I usually _____

If I think I will stutter in the classroom, I usually _____

If I could tell my classmates one thing about my speech, it would be _____

_____

_____

Answer the following questions.

	Yes	No	Sometimes
I like reading out loud in school.	____	____	____
I raise my hand when I know the answer.	____	____	____
If I have something to say, I say it no matter what.	____	____	____
If I think I might stutter, I may not say anything.	____	____	____
The other children in my class are okay with my speech.	____	____	____
I think my teacher knows a lot about stuttering.	____	____	____
I get teased about my speech (now or in the past).	____	____	____
I know a lot about stuttering.	____	____	____

Overall Evaluation Summary

Child's Name _____ Age/Grade _____ Date of Evaluation _____

Relevant Speech/Language and Medical History

Medical History	Other Communication Disorders	Prior Treatment History

Observable Characteristics of Stuttering *(based on observation of multiple speech samples)*

Disfluency Characteristics

Situation	Stutt.	Nonstutt.
	%	%
	%	%

Common Types _____

Avg. Duration _____

Overall Severity _____

Related Behaviors *(check all that apply, add others as necessary)*

___ eye blinks/poor eye contact   ___ voice tension/rising pitch

___ facial tension or struggle   ___ body movements

___ other (_____)

Physical Characteristics of Stuttering

Child's Reactions to Stuttering *(based on interview, standardized tests, and portfolio assessment)*

Beliefs About Stuttering

Feelings About Stuttering

Avoidance Reactions

___ refusing to speak/not answering questions

___ having others speak for him/her

___ circumlocution/changing words/avoiding words

___ using fillers or starter words and sounds

___ other (_____)

Child's Speech/Language Development *(based on standardized tests, observation parent/teacher reports)*

Vocabulary/Word Retrieval

Syntax

Articulation/Phonology

Oral-Motor Skills

Voice

Other People's Reactions to Stuttering

Parents	**Teachers**	**Peers/Siblings/Others**
Beliefs & Feelings	Beliefs & Feelings	Beliefs & Feelings
Level of Concern	Level of Concern	Reactions
Expectations & Goals	Expectations & Goals	

Suggested Outline of Initial Parent Conference ———————

1. **Introduction**

   o Review Referral Source/Purpose of Evaluation

   o Review Relevant Case History

   o Initial Discussion of the Nature and Cause of Stuttering

2. **Presentation of Findings**

   o Describe Evaluation Process

   o Review *Overall Evaluation Summary* form

   - Observable Characteristics of Stuttering
     (include explanation of terminology)

   - Child's Reactions to Stuttering

   - Child's Speech and Language Development

   - Other People's Reactions to Stuttering

3. **Discuss Treatment Recommendations**

   o Consider Eligibility and Placement

   o Create Goals and Benchmarks
     (with input from assessment team, including parents and teachers)

Appendix 3M
The Source for School-Age Stuttering

116

Copyright © 2003 LinguiSystems, Inc.

Suggested Outline of Follow-Up Conference

1. **Review *Parent Questionnaire* and *Case History* forms.**

   o Request additional information or clarification about parents' perceptions and child's experiences.

   o Answer parents' questions arising from forms or initial parent conference.

2. **Discuss nature of stuttering.**

   o Dispel myths about stuttering (causes, treatment goals, parent responsibility, etc.).

   o Explain the difference between observable speech behaviors (disfluencies) and the overall stuttering disorder.

   o Educate parents about the connection between affective, behavioral, and cognitive components of stuttering.

   o Review internal and external factors that may contribute to speech disruptions.

   o Emphasize the variability of stuttering behaviors (explain that there are "easy days" and "harder days") and review factors that may influence this variability.

3. **Review short-term and long-term goals of treatment.**

4. **Explain process of therapy.**

   o Describe therapy activities, expectations for child, home practice routines, etc.

   o Highlight value and roles of the child's "team" (family, clinician, teacher, others).

5. **Answer additional questions.**

6. **Establish procedures for on-going contact.**

   o Review parent involvement in therapy.

   o Schedule follow-up parent interactions.

   o Plan visits to therapy sessions.

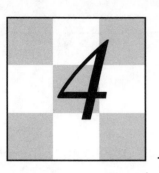

He Needs Treatment — Now What?

Doesn't He Just Need to Slow Down and Take a Deep Breath?

There are many myths and misconceptions about stuttering (Bloodstein 1993). One of the side-effects of these misunderstandings among clinicians, and in society in general, is the fact that many different therapy ideas have been proposed. Some of these therapy ideas are valuable, for they are based on clinical experience and data-based evidence. Others, unfortunately, are not. As clinicians who understand stuttering, it is your responsibility to educate others about this disorder, the intricate nature of stuttering therapy, and the long-term implications of dealing with a stuttering disorder.

Myth: There is one best way to treat stuttering.

One of the most common myths in the field of speech-language pathology is the idea that there is one "best" way to treat stuttering. This notion may come from a decades-long history of "one size fits all" treatments. It often seems that researchers or clinicians experienced some success with a particular client and, as a result, suggest that their particular treatment approach should be effective for *every* person who stutters. Fortunately, we now know that stuttering is much too complex and variable to be treated in only one way. Different people have different needs in therapy, and different approaches work for different people. Thus, individualized treatment plans are the only way to successfully help people who stutter achieve their optimal outcome from therapy. In other words, clinicians must learn to fit their therapy to the child, rather than trying to fit the child to the therapy.

Of course, we recognize that what we are writing about in this book can also be considered just "one way" of treating stuttering. Indeed, this is true! While we know that the framework we are presenting in this book can be helpful for many children who stutter, we also believe there are other treatment approaches that clinicians should consider. Just as we do not want other clinicians to promote their approaches as the only way of treating stuttering, we, too, do not want to suggest that our way is the only way. We strongly encourage you to learn as much about stuttering as possible, including various philosophies and methods of treatment.

"Canned" treatments cannot apply to everybody.

Because stuttering is highly variable and complex, and because children who stutter are such a heterogeneous group, strictly programmed approaches to therapy cannot work equally well for all children. We hope that when you have finished reading this book, and when you have gained some experience with the varied and integrated treatment methods we describe, you will recognize that we are presenting a multi-faceted, problem-solving approach to stuttering therapy that allows the flexibility that is needed for working with different individuals.

In this chapter, we have tried to provide enough detail about this treatment so that you will be able to understand the philosophy behind the treatment and apply the methods we use on a daily basis with children who stutter. At the same time, however, we have tried not to present this approach as a "canned" program with simplistic "step-by-step" instructions. Our primary goal is to present therapy ideas and strategies that will empower you to use your own knowledge, problem-solving skills, and clinical judgment. We hope that the information we include will support you in expanding your existing skills and that the resources we provide will help you stretch even further to improve your skills for the benefit of children who stutter.

The parents have just heard of a "better" approach.

From time to time, we all hear about so-called "new" or "better" treatments for stuttering. These may include new techniques, medications, or even electronic devices that are supposed to reduce or eliminate stuttering. Often, these treatments sound too good to be true, and in many cases, they are.

Unfortunately, hopeful parents and family members may be tempted by the promise of a cure or a new, slick advertising campaign that makes it sound like their child will finally be able to overcome his stuttering once and for all. Some advertisements may even attempt to capitalize on parents' feelings of guilt about whether they are doing enough to help their child. The appeal of such promises is not hard to understand — it can be difficult for families to accept their child's stuttering, and it is definitely difficult for the child to change his stuttering—so it is not surprising that these claims may catch parents' attention.

Ideally, when a parent hears of a new technique or treatment, he or she will come to you to ask for more information. We say "ideally" because we view this as an excellent opportunity to educate the parents about the true nature of stuttering. Children who stutter and their families will be faced with promises of "miracle cures" all their lives, and they need to learn how to distinguish between real treatment opportunities and approaches that offer little more than false hope. Thus, rather than seeing this situation as a challenge to your clinical skills or knowledge, use this situation to your advantage in your efforts to help the child and support the parents.

In some cases, the information the parents have uncovered may indeed represent an advance in the treatment of stuttering. Therefore, you should be sure to listen carefully to what they present and work with them to evaluate the appropriateness of a potentially new approach. In addition to demonstrating your interest in their child's well-being, this meeting will provide you with the opportunity to develop a greater understanding of the factors that may improve the child's ability to communicate.

We hasten to add, however, that such explorations should be based on a solid understanding of the nature of stuttering. We have known too many clinicians who, like the hopeful parents, were drawn in by promises of easier treatment and greater success. Some have tried novel approaches simply because they did not truly understand the approach they were already using. Therefore, we prefer to take an attitude of cautious optimism when we hear about new treatment options. We are always interested to learn about new ways of helping people who stutter, though we have seen many examples of new treatments that turned out to be "old wine in new bottles" or cures that were based on faulty evidence or no evidence at all. By combining your clinical judgment, your understanding of stuttering (derived from several sources), and your relationship with the child and family, you will be able to help the parents make appropriate decisions about their child's treatment.

Why are there so many techniques?

Clinicians who are beginning to expand their knowledge about stuttering often wonder why there are so many different approaches for treating stuttering. There are a number of reasons for this diversity of opinion and thought about stuttering therapy.

First, as we have established previously, stuttering is a multi-faceted disorder, and what you see is not always what you get. When individual researchers and clinicians have approached the problem of stuttering, they have, necessarily, approached it from their own particular bias or perspective. As a result, they have highlighted or focused their efforts on those aspects of the disorder that were most important in their own framework. Because of this, different approaches seem to work for some people but not for others. This suggests that clinicians can gain the greatest appreciation for the stuttering disorder if they embrace many different perspectives and try to find the factors that seem to apply to each individual person who stutters.

Another key factor contributing to the differences of opinion on stuttering treatment is the simple fact that every person who stutters is different from every other person who stutters. Again, what works for one person will not necessarily work the same way for another person. Just as there are several different approaches for treating articulation, language, voice, and swallowing disorders, there is more than one way to treat stuttering. If we keep in mind the fact that the approaches we learn will only apply to a certain percentage of people who stutter, then we can develop an array of different strategies for helping different people rather than trying to fit everybody we work with into a particular mold.

Unfortunately, it seems that the large number of options for helping people who stutter has been viewed by some as a roadblock to learning about stuttering rather than as an opportunity to draw from a variety of helpful perspectives. It is our hope that you will come to see the diversity of opinions about stuttering treatment as one of the strengths of this field rather than as a weakness.

Which theory is right?

Along with the differences in treatment approaches, there is a staggering array of current and historical theories about stuttering. Indeed, in the history of the study of stuttering, there have been periods of significant theory development and speculation. (See reviews in Bloodstein 1993, 1995). Some of the theories about stuttering that have been developed were directly tied to a specific therapeutic approach, while others were not. Like the different therapy approaches mentioned above, however, these different theories were all based on the particular frameworks or philosophies of the specific researchers or clinicians who developed them. Thus, each is necessarily incomplete. Though there has been significant progress made in the past several years aimed at taking a more broad-based and comprehensive view of stuttering (Conture 2001, Smith & Kelly 1997, Starkweather & Givens-Ackerman 1997), there is still no single theory that adequately explains all aspects of stuttering.

Sadly, many clinicians report to us that the only thing they remember about the stuttering class they had during their graduate training is the fact that there are many theories about stuttering and that none of the experts agree with one another! For some, this can lead to a feeling of frustration or hopelessness about one's ability to understand stuttering well enough to become an expert clinician, and it has discouraged many clinicians from developing their interest in stuttering.

In our opinion, it is not really necessary for you to have a detailed knowledge of all of the theories about stuttering that have been proposed in the literature over the years. Certainly, you do not want to be ignorant of history. At the same time, however, you also do not want your concerns about learning the literature to keep you from focusing on developing clinical skills based on current understandings of the disorder.

In the end, we believe that people who stutter will be best served when clinicians develop a broad-based understanding of stuttering that draws upon key elements from several different theories. This is the type of understanding we are attempting to present in this book. We strongly encourage you to supplement the information gained from this volume with knowledge from many other sources, including other books on stuttering, information presented by experts in this field, your own clinical work, and the wisdom and experience gained from listening to people who stutter.

It's Not a Cookbook

Learning to handle a stuttering problem can be a long-term process, and children who stutter must be allowed to take their own time and follow their own courses. Your job is to be their guide, to show them the choices that are available to them, and then to walk the paths with them. Eventually, however, the children we serve must choose their own paths.

Inherent in this philosophy is the belief that there is no specific destination or outcome that is required for all individuals. Thus, we believe that success should not be defined simply as the moment when a child reaches an arbitrarily chosen target (e.g., "less than 2% syllables stuttered" or "normal fluency"). As we will explain in more detail, our broad-based philosophy about the nature of treatment can make documentation of treatment outcomes more challenging. Still, it is not impossible. If we are to help children who stutter, we must not limit ourselves only to those areas of treatment that are easily measured (i.e., too much concentration on percentages and targets). We can be highly effective clinicians when we help children set broad-based goals, support them as they move toward achieving those goals, and problem solve with them to adjust the goals when necessary.

We must become our own "problem solvers" and "critical thinkers."

Throughout their lives, children who stutter will encounter many different situations and experiences. If they are to overcome the challenges they face, they will need to develop the abilities to examine problems objectively, consider different solutions, and select options that give them the best opportunities for success.

To help them develop the skills they will need, we must be certain that children understand the necessity of becoming independent problem solvers. From the initial assessment, throughout daily intervention, to the conclusion of treatment, they must feel that they are an integral part of their own treatment plans. Children must understand that they are directly responsible for their success. At the same time, they must recognize that they are not "failing" when therapy hits a snag. They must become adept at examining challenging situations, and they must be able to use critical thinking skills to identify solutions and incorporate changes into their daily lives to help them achieve success. The ultimate goal is for children to become their own speech clinicians so they can continue the lifelong process of improving their speech even after the formal treatment period has ended.

We can help children become more active participants in their own therapies through the example we provide. We are a key role model for showing children how to apply problem-solving skills in the development and use of an individualized therapy plan. By including children in the day-to-day process of planning and implementing therapy, we can show them how we make decisions about what goals to pursue in therapy, and what strategies to employ to achieve those goals. As we involve children in the discussion about these goals and strategies, we can help them develop a sense of ownership in their therapies that will ultimately help them play a more active role in their treatment.

One way we can help children understand the stages involved in problem solving is to draw upon models used by social workers and psychologists. For example, variations of the following seven steps appear fairly consistently in various models from the literature on problem solving (e.g., Egan 2002):

1. Identify the problem.
2. Brainstorm possible solutions.
3. Discuss consequences of each identified solution.
4. Categorize solutions to narrow the list of potential options.
5. Choose one option and create a plan of action.
6. Follow the action plan and examine the outcome.
7. Try again if the solution does not produce a desirable result.

We can adapt this model in creating a more "child-friendly" version that can help our young students feel more comfortable with the problem-solving process:

1. Name it.
2. Drain your brain.
3. Look ahead.
4. Group 'em.
5. Pick one and plan it.
6. Try it and rate it.
7. Do-overs allowed.

By encouraging children to engage in these types of problem-solving activities, and by incorporating problem-solving opportunities into therapy on a daily basis, you can help children develop the skills they will need to overcome the challenges they face both in and out of therapy. The plan sheet in Appendix 4A, page 179 can be used with a child to help him come up with his own problem-solving plan. A completed example of a plan sheet can be found in Chapter 7, Appendix 7A, page 274.

Therapy must be based on principles, not programs.

In the previous sections, we emphasized two facts: First, every child is different, so you must develop individualized treatment programs that meet the specific needs of each child you work with. Second, you and your students must become problem solvers who can identify novel solutions to the challenges they face, both in therapy and beyond.

Together, these two points have one important implication: both you and your students must understand *why* you are doing the things you are doing in therapy. Without a thorough understanding of the principles behind therapy, you will be unable to adapt the treatment to each child's needs, and your children will be unable to apply the knowledge and skills gained in the therapy room to other situations they face.

Developing individualized therapy approaches that are based on sound principles rather than a prepackaged program has many advantages. First, if you understand the rationale behind the treatment strategies, you will have more confidence in your clinical skills, and you will be better able to incorporate new knowledge and evaluate new approaches to treatment. Even more importantly, children who understand the principles behind their therapy goals and strategies will feel more motivated in therapy, and they will take more responsibility for improving their own communication skills. Furthermore, children who understand why they are doing the things they are doing in therapy will be more likely to generalize their strategies to new situations and, ultimately, maintain their success over time.

Helping children understand the rationale behind the therapy is not simply a matter of repeatedly telling them why they are doing things. Of course, when we introduce a new strategy or concept, we need to discuss with the child the reasons we are doing that activity or addressing that topic. Beyond that, however, we must continue to review the rationale for treatment with the child throughout the therapy process. When speech tools are practiced or when various issues are discussed, we must review the rationale. We prefer to do this, not by teaching or lecturing the child, but by *asking the child* to explain the rationale to us or to another person (e.g., a peer or parent). This type of reflective therapy provides children with numerous opportunities to solidify their understanding of the rationale for treatment while reinforcing the lessons we are trying to teach.

Choosing the Direction of Therapy

One of the first decisions that must be made in the early stages of therapy is specifically what direction the therapy will take. In Chapter 3, we discussed a number of issues that need to be addressed regarding the recommendation of treatment. Now, we must make specific decisions about what the child will do in therapy.

Who decides?

Typically, a child is brought to your attention because somebody in the child's environment has noticed a concern with his speech. Perhaps the teacher has noticed a problem in the classroom, or perhaps the parent has alerted you to an existing problem in the child's speech. In some cases, it may actually be the child himself who has sought out the treatment. However, more often than not, there is somebody in the child's support system who has identified the problem and sought treatment. As described in Chapter 3, following this referral, an evaluation is conducted and recommendations are made about the appropriateness of treatment at a particular point in time. Various members of the support team may then meet in an IEP meeting or parent counseling session and, if warranted, the child's treatment is scheduled.

All of this is as it should be; the people in the child's environment are working together to ensure the best possible treatment situation for the child. Any experienced clinician will know, however, that this does not necessarily mean that the child will achieve the outcome that the support team envisioned or hoped for. Simply recommending, initiating, and conducting treatment does not guarantee success. Ultimately, the responsibility for change falls to the child, and all of the encouragement, support, and persuasion will not convince a child to make changes in his speech if he is not ready.

This means that the support team must listen to the child to learn about his interest in therapy, his motivation for making changes in his speech, and his willingness to use those modifications both in and out of therapy. Thus, although the members of the child's support team provide input into the treatment plan, and although you and the parents play a major role in determining this course of treatment, you must also work within the boundaries of what the child is willing or able to do. You can serve as a guide and companion, but the child has the ultimate choice of how and when he wants to work through the process of dealing with his stuttering.

How direct can I get?

Often we are asked how "direct" you should get when working with young children who stutter. The question probably arises because many clinicians are familiar with so-called "indirect" therapy approaches that are often used with *preschool* children (not school-age) who stutter.

The fundamental definition of indirect approaches for preschool children is that they do not specifically require the child to exhibit specific changes in their speech during therapy (Conture 2001, Guitar 1998). Instead, they focus on eliciting the desired changes through modeling (i.e., showing the child the correct form) and other strategies designed to encourage the child to change his speaking pattern on his own, without direct correction from the clinician.

There is, at present, a significant debate in the field of fluency disorders about the value of indirect therapy approaches for preschoolers who stutter (Nippold & Rudzinski 1995). Presumably, these approaches were developed because of clinicians' concerns that overtly correcting a child's speech or drawing attention to stuttering might in some way make the child's stuttering worse. Today, we know that simply talking about stuttering does not necessarily have a negative impact on a child's speech (Logan & Yaruss 1999, Harris et al. 2002). Still, many clinicians continue to be reluctant to engage in more direct therapy approaches with very young children.

When we are working with *school-age* children, however, the situation is much different. By the time a child reaches the school-age years, he is most certainly aware of his stuttering. Attention has already been drawn to his speech, either by himself or by others, and the chances are good that he has already tried various ways of changing the way he talks. For school-age children, therefore, it makes little sense for clinicians to use an indirect therapy approach that is designed to avoid drawing attention to or talking about stuttering.

Therefore, we almost always use a direct approach when working with school-age children who stutter. This does not mean that we use harsh, direct criticism of the child's speech. It simply means that we do not shy away from talking about speech and working specifically on the child's stuttering and overall communication patterns. Because we use individualized therapy approaches for each of the children we work with, we recognize that different children will require different strategies and different degrees of directness. Still, for school-age children, nearly all of the work we do would be considered direct therapy.

Of course, in determining how direct to be in therapy, we must also follow the child's lead and incorporate discussions about stuttering, fluency management techniques, and acceptance of stuttering at a level that is appropriate for the child's degree of readiness at that time. Sometimes, if a child is not ready to address a certain goal, we can focus our attention on other goals, or work on leading up to the desired goal in a gradual, supportive fashion that takes the child's needs and capabilities into account. In this way, we can design individualized therapy programs that help children reach the goals that are most important to them at a particular time and that have the greatest chance of achieving success over the long term.

Treating stuttering doesn't mean just treating "stuttering"

Throughout this book, we have emphasized the importance of taking a broad-based view of the stuttering disorder, and, ultimately, of adopting a broad-based approach to treatment. This means that treating the child's stuttering does not just mean working on his speech behaviors and assuming that the rest of the disorder will take care of itself.

In the next section, we outline the specific components of a comprehensive treatment approach. Because every child is different, we do not necessarily do all of these things with every child we see. Still, these are the primary areas we consider as we develop an individualized treatment plan for a school-age child who stutters.

Setting the Stage for Therapy

Before we can begin helping the child improve his fluency, his attitudes about his stuttering, and his communication abilities, there is a considerable amount of background information he must learn about speaking, about stuttering, and about communication in general. Thus, at the outset of treatment, we work with the child to "set the stage" and provide a solid foundation for success in treatment.

Speech notebook

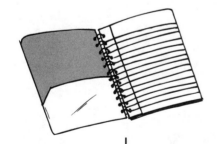

The first activity in therapy is the selection and preparation of the child's "speech notebook." The primary purpose of the speech notebook is to give the child a central place where he can record his experiences, thoughts, feelings, drawings, questions, and skill-building activities so he can review them as he progresses through treatment.

The notebook also serves several other purposes. It helps to foster a sense of ownership in therapy for the child so he can develop a record of all of the things he has done to help himself with his speech. It also provides the child with an easy way of "going back to the basics" when he is learning how to independently face challenges and solve problems he experiences both in and out of therapy. An added bonus is the fact that the notebook is actually a form of portfolio-based documentation that provides a helpful means of measuring progress in therapy and changes in the child's speech and communication attitudes over time.

The "speech notebook" is simple and flexible—it can be whatever the child wants to create. Everyone in the child's environment can share their thoughts in the pages of the child's speech notebook. Ultimately, the notebook provides a visual representation of the child's journey through therapy.

After the child has prepared his speech notebook, he is ready to start filling it with important information about speaking, stuttering, and communicating. This is the information that will provide the foundation for his success in treatment.

Learning about speech

For most people, speaking is an automatic activity. Typically fluent children and adults speak almost effortlessly, smoothly planning what they want to say without thinking about whether they will be able to say it. People who stutter, on the other hand, may spend a great deal of time and effort thinking about the way they talk. They may focus on the physical sensations of tension and struggle they experience during moments of stuttering or they may focus on the emotional reactions to the stuttering, such as the anxiety and fear associated with listeners' reactions to stuttering (Williams 1957).

That said, neither people who stutter nor typically fluent speakers have a very detailed understanding of what actually happens with their speech mechanisms while they are talking. They are largely unaware of the intricate link between anatomical structures such as the lungs and rib cage, the larynx, and the mouth. And, they may have very little concept of what is actually involved in planning and producing speech. For most people, this is not a problem, for they do not need to think about how they speak in order to communicate easily and successfully.

For people who stutter, the lack of understanding about speech production can be a hindrance to success in speech therapy. It can also contribute to ongoing attempts to modify speech that actually do more harm than good. Therefore, one of the first, most important steps in therapy is to help the child learn more about the process of speaking (Williams 1957, 1971).

Understanding the "speech machine"

The first thing the child needs to learn is what parts of the body are involved in producing speech (Guitar 1998, Ramig & Bennett 1997). Teaching the child about the speech production process involves much more than just showing him diagrams of anatomy and explaining how the respiratory, phonatory, and articulatory systems work. Ideally, the child will develop an understanding of how his speech mechanism functions through *exploration*. As you know, it is easier to engage a child's interest in difficult tasks if you adjust the task to his level of interest and ability. For example, two of the most useful tools for bringing complicated topics to a child's cognitive level are drawing and building. You can use these types of activities to help children learn about their speech.

1. Begin by simply asking the child what parts of his body he uses for speaking. You can also ask questions like "What's the very first thing you do when you want to say something?" and "What is the next thing you do?"

   We are often surprised by the insights children share when their attention is drawn to different parts of the speech production mechanism. By asking questions like "What is going on in your mouth right now?" or "What is your tongue doing?", you can help children focus on different parts of the speaking process so they can begin to understand what their bodies are doing during both fluent and stuttered speech.

2. Have the child draw the various parts of his body that he uses when he speaks. You can trace the child's outline on a large sheet of paper or the child can draw a smaller representation in his speech notebook. Help the child fill in and identify key parts of the respiratory system (e.g., diaphragm, lungs, ribs, abdominal muscles) using colored pencils or crayons. You can show him the different positions these body parts are in during quiet breathing and during speech breathing.

   You can do the same thing to show him what happens when he is producing voice by drawing a model of the throat, including structures such as the larynx and vocal folds. For younger children, this can be adapted so the list of structures is more straightforward (e.g., mouth, voice box, lungs). Regardless of your students' levels of cognitive development, you can select terms they can use to gain a better understanding of what is going on in their bodies when they are speaking.

Remember, the child's drawings and models do not have to be sophisticated or artistic (and neither do yours). They simply need to reflect the key anatomical components in the speech production system and demonstrate the important physiological relationships between these subsystems. This will help the child have a visual picture of what is going on inside his body when he is speaking. In addition to giving the child a frame of reference when he is exploring different ways of talking, it will also help him develop an appropriate vocabulary that he can use when learning about speech.

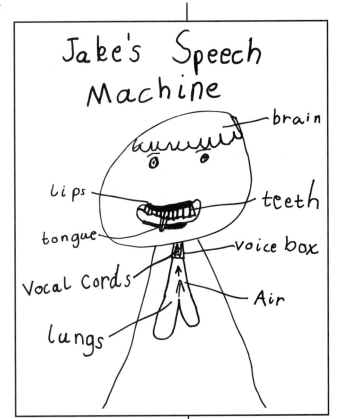

3. Have the child make a model using clay or Legos to represent the speech production subsystems.

4. Help the child see how voice is produced by folding a piece of paper in half and blowing across the edge of it to demonstrate how the vocal folds work. The rapid vibration and "clapping together" of the sheets of paper will make a sound similar in many ways to the sound generated by the vocal folds.

5. Have the child identify the lips, teeth, hard and soft palate, and tongue as key structures that move together to produce the sounds of speech. The child can experiment with producing different sounds and different combinations of movement to understand how speech is produced.

6. Finally, explain how all of these parts of the body work together during communication. For example, you might say "The brain tells all the other parts of the speech machine what to do. First, the lungs take in the air. When we push the air out, that makes the vocal cords vibrate. The sound from the vocal cords travels up to the mouth. Inside the mouth, we move the tongue and lips in various ways to make different sounds." Of course, the specific terminology can be adjusted to the child's level of development

and individual preferences. Some children will enjoy learning terminology like "larynx" and "vocal folds" while others will be more comfortable talking about the "voice box."

Ask Ourselves: Why Are We Doing This?

We cannot change what we do not understand. Thus, a working knowledge of the speech system is an essential first step for children who wish to make changes in their speech. You can guide children through the basics of speech anatomy and physiology, and this will help to make the speaking process easier for the child to understand. Exploring this piece of the puzzle with children of all ages is not only critical, it's fun! Many children are highly motivated to learn the "science" behind their speech, for developing a sense of expertise about speaking and stuttering can help them feel less afraid of their speech and less likely to be embarrassed about their stuttering.

By making "speech machines" or "speech people," children can explore the ways their physiological subsystems work together when they speak (Guitar 1998, Ramig & Bennett 1997). Such activities can easily be scaled so they are appropriate for the child's age, language ability, and vocabulary. Regardless of the child's age, however, we always seek to teach the child as much as we can about his speech mechanisms.

Tuning in to speech

There are many ways children can develop an increased understanding about speaking:

- learn about the speech machine
- watch other people speaking
- listen to different ways of talking
- explore different choices for talking (e.g., pitch, loudness, rate)
- observe a visual representation of speech using a system like *VisiPitch* from Kay Elemetrics
- focus on their own speech and try to sense what their articulators are doing

By "tuning in" to their own speech and by focusing on the proprioceptive feedback they receive from the tongue, cheeks, jaw, and throat, children can begin to learn more about how their mouths move during both fluent speech and stuttering. By paying more attention to proprioception, and by talking about their observations with you, children improve their understanding of how different parts of their mouths work together. They will learn how the different parts of their bodies are used for talking and how they are linked together as speech is produced.

Playing with Speech

Children can also increase their understanding of the speech process by "playing with their speech," or talking in different ways (e.g., using a high voice, using a low voice, speaking faster, speaking slower, stretching out speech, increasing or decreasing pausing). All of these speech changes help the child "set the stage" for the later introduction of strategies designed to increase fluency or change physical tension during moments of stuttering (Quesal & Yaruss 2000, Williams 1971).

Note that activities for playing with speech are not themselves focused on increasing fluency. They also are not the same as oral-motor exercises, which may be designed to strengthen the child's oral structures or improve coordination (Riley & Riley 1985). They are simply an opportunity for the child to become more comfortable talking about talking, moving the mouth for speech, and talking in new and different ways. All of these are skills the child will need in order to become successful at making the specific types of speech changes being addressed in therapy (Williams 1971).

Learning about stuttering

People who stutter do not enjoy stuttering. For many speakers, the experience of being "stuck" in a block is one of the most uncomfortable feelings they know. You can experience a little bit of this same discomfort yourself by simply trying a little "pseudo-stuttering" or stuttering on purpose, in real-world situations. Feelings of embarrassment, anxiety about what other people are thinking, and the fear that the word may never come out can be extreme. As a result, many people who stutter try their best *not* to think about what is happening with their speech during a moment of stuttering. Some even report that they "tune out" during stuttering so they don't have to feel the full effect of the discomfort associated with being in a moment of stuttering (Van Riper 1982).

For this reason, many children who stutter may not have a detailed awareness of what they do when they stutter. For example, they may not actually be aware of the facial movements, breathing irregularities, or physical gestures they exhibit in blocks. Of course, some speakers are acutely aware of these observable features of their stuttering, and this may actually serve to increase their fear about stuttering. Even so, children who stutter may not have an adequate understanding of the stuttering moments themselves. Therefore, just as it is necessary to educate children who stutter about the speech mechanism and the way they use their respiratory, phonatory, and articulatory systems to produce speech, it is also necessary to educate children who stutter about stuttering. Later in this chapter, we talk about specific strategies for helping children who stutter learn about their stuttering.

Getting the facts

At appropriate ages and levels of awareness, children need to learn the facts about stuttering (or "bumpy speech" or "stuck speech" or whatever the child feels comfortable calling his disfluencies). We can start by providing facts about the types of disfluencies speakers produce and explain the difference between stuttering and normal disfluencies. We can also help the child learn about the prevalence of stuttering, current ideas about the cause of stuttering, and different approaches to the treatment of stuttering.

As with all other aspects of therapy, the child will learn best if he is encouraged to develop his understanding of these key facts on his own rather than just receiving the information in the form of a handout or lecture. This does not mean that the child has to do all this work by himself. You and the child can work together to research information about stuttering using sources such as textbooks, the Internet, and information available from groups such as the Stuttering Foundation of America (SFA) or the National Stuttering Association (NSA).

We can also help children learn more about their own stuttering through fun activities that create a positive awareness of what happens during moments of stuttering. Just as we help children learn about their speech machines and how they work to produce fluent speech, we also help them examine the tension that they experience in moments of stuttering.

Can I say the "s" word?

Sometimes, people in the child's environment may have tried to avoid saying the word *stuttering* in front of the child. The reasons for this are varied; however, it probably dates back to the time when parents were encouraged not to draw attention to a child's stuttering in an apparent attempt to prevent the negative reactions that characterize stuttering. Today, however, we know that talking about stuttering does not necessarily make children feel bad about their speech. In fact, if done appropriately, talking about stuttering can actually help children come to terms with their speaking difficulties (Logan & Yaruss 1999, Starkweather & Givens-Ackerman 1997).

Thus, we do not hesitate to use the word *stuttering* when talking with children about their speech. We want children to recognize that it is not the *word* itself that is problematic but the stigma that society has attached to this word that makes some people uncomfortable with the word *stuttering*. We know that children are going to hear this word from other people, so we want to make sure that they are not embarrassed or uncomfortable when they hear people mention stuttering.

Even though we feel free to talk about stuttering with children, we also feel that it is a good idea to use the specific label that the child uses to describe his stuttering (e.g., bumpy, tight). Particularly with younger children, or with children who are new to therapy, we begin by asking questions such as, "What are some words people can use to talk about tension in talking?" Many times, this leads to a list that *includes* the word *stuttering*, thereby making it just another word that is used to label what is happening with the child's speech. By helping the child develop a vocabulary for talking about stuttering in an open, honest, matter-of-fact way, we can help to minimize the stigma and reduce the power that any one particular word may have over him.

Tight and loose

One aspect of speech production that is particularly important for children who stutter to understand is the role of physical tension. During moments of stuttering—and even during seemingly fluent speech—the muscles involved in speech production are often tensed too tightly (Williams 1971). It may also be that opposing muscle groups may be tensed in opposition to each other, resulting in co-contraction (Gilman & Yaruss 2000). The result is that the child feels stuck, like he cannot move his mouth or tongue during the moment of the block.

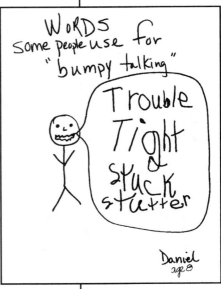

Ultimately, our goal will be to teach children to reduce excess tension in the muscles that are involved in a moment of stuttering. This will play an important role in the development of strategies for modifying stuttering. In the early stages of treatment, however, we may simply need to introduce the proprioceptive difference between physically tense muscles and physically relaxed muscles. (Though this may seem obvious to you, it is not necessarily obvious to the child.) Children need to understand that a certain amount of physical tension is necessary for speech—tensing of muscles in and of itself is not a bad thing. Too much tension makes it difficult to speak smoothly, but too little tension is also a problem (Conture 2001).

To help children learn the difference between *tensed* and *relaxed* muscles and to help them learn to modify the tension in their speech, we can engage in a variety of therapy activities that highlight physical tension. One activity involves asking the child to "tense up" different parts of his body, hold onto that tension, and then relax that tension when asked. Children usually find this activity to be quite fun. You and the child can take turns asking each other to tense up and relax your feet, your hands, your heads, your noses, and, ultimately, your lips, your tongue, your voice box, your abdomen, and other parts of the body used for speech (Dell 1993). Another effective strategy is to have the child throw a soft ball or crumpled up piece of paper at the wall while his arm is relaxed and again when his arm is very tense. When the child's arm is very tense, the ball rarely makes it to the wall before hitting the ground. When the child's arm is relaxed, the ball goes much closer to the intended target.

Recall that the goal of these exercises is not to get the child relaxed, calm, or fluent. Instead, the goal is to teach the child how muscles feel when they have too much or too little physical tension. A second, equally important goal is to teach the child that he *can* modify the amount of tension in his muscles. Thus, even if the child is in a fairly tense moment of stuttering, he can, with practice, learn to reduce that tension so the moment of stuttering is not as severe, as long, or as uncomfortable. We will say more about how to introduce these stuttering modification strategies later in this chapter. For now, however, the focus is on teaching the child that he *can* learn to reduce excess tension in his speech muscles.

Ask Ourselves: Is the Child Ready for This?

We often hear clinicians ask whether a child is "ready" for a certain aspect of therapy. The answer, unfortunately, is that it is not always easy to tell. Some children will progress through therapy quite rapidly, while others will need more time for different stages of treatment. The older the child is, the easier it is to gauge readiness. If you have developed an open dialogue with the child about talking, stuttering, and speech therapy, you can and should ask the child how he is feeling about various topics being addressed in treatment (e.g., "How are we doing in therapy?" "How does this seem to you?" "Is this a good goal for you?").

For younger children, or for older children who are less willing to provide feedback and play an active role in guiding treatment, it may be harder to tell if they are moving along at the right pace. As a result, it may be necessary for you to try different strategies or

continued

goals and see how the child responds. Often, it becomes very clear when a child is not ready to address a certain goal or use a specific strategy. In such cases, you should adapt therapy accordingly so the child can achieve success with a different, more appropriate goal.

There are two key issues you should keep in mind when evaluating the child's readiness for therapy goals. First, remember that therapy for stuttering takes time. A child may go weeks or months without making noticeable progress on a particular goal, even if he is working hard and is motivated to achieve success. The strategies we ask children to learn and the changes we are asking them to make in therapy can be quite difficult. Furthermore, by the time a child has reached the school-age years, speaking and stuttering patterns have become quite entrenched. Thus, it may take some children quite a bit of time to achieve mastery of new speaking skills.

Second, particularly when you are addressing affective and cognitive aspects of stuttering, keep in mind that many children *will* be uncomfortable with certain therapy activities when they are first introduced. The topics we bring up in speech therapy for children who stutter are not easy to talk about; if they were easy, then the child would probably not need therapy to deal with them. (Certainly, if a child is not experiencing negative affective or cognitive reactions to stuttering, then you do not need to address them in therapy.)

If a child is experiencing negative reactions to his stuttering, it is likely that he will express some discomfort or reluctance when you begin to address these new, difficult topics. You should not allow the child's discomfort to prevent you from addressing issues in therapy that must be addressed. Of course, this does not mean that you need to force a child to talk about things that make him uncomfortable. Still, if negative emotional reactions are affecting a child's ability to communicate or impeding progress in therapy, it is important to address them in a supportive fashion even if the child is initially reluctant to do so. If a child does not want to talk about stuttering on the first day of therapy, the topic shouldn't be discarded for the duration of therapy. Instead, you may wish to introduce the topic gradually over several sessions and work to minimize the child's concerns along the way.

You must learn the difference between *reluctance*, or the natural reticence people may exhibit when talking about something that is uncomfortable for them, and *resistance*, the stronger, more oppositional "pushing back" that people may exhibit when asked to talk about something that they are not ready or willing to talk about (Egan 2002). By carefully considering whether the child is exhibiting reluctance or resistance, you can judge whether it is appropriate to set a new topic aside until the child is ready, or whether it is appropriate to continue the discussion in a gentle, supportive way, while acknowledging the fact that dealing with stuttering is not always easy to do.

Discussing relaxation techniques

You are probably familiar with relaxation techniques that are designed to help the child who stutters "relax." On the surface, the use of relaxation techniques may seem to make sense, since children who stutter often exhibit excess physical tension in their speech (Gregory 2003). Some children may even seem to be nervous or uptight due to their anxiety about speaking and stuttering. Therefore, over the years, clinicians have introduced various techniques for helping people who stutter relax their muscles (Gilman & Yaruss 2000). Some of these strategies have included not only the muscles involved in speaking, but also the muscles of the entire body.

An example of this is seen with "progressive relaxation" exercises in which a person is asked to tense and relax individual parts of the body, beginning with the feet and legs, then gradually work his way through the torso, arms, neck, face, and oral articulators (Jacobson 1938, Wolpe 1958). The use of such relaxation techniques in stuttering therapy dates back roughly 200 years (Gilman & Yaruss 2000). Following a progressive relaxation exercise, the speaker is supposed to be more relaxed overall, and this relaxation is then supposed to translate into easier, more fluent speech. Ultimately, practitioners who use such approaches believe that the child will learn to generalize this feeling of relaxation to other settings through visualization or direct practice so he can relax in situations where he feels anxiety. Supposedly, this reduction in anxiety will translate to increased fluency. You are probably able to tell from reading this paragraph that the situation is not quite that simple.

There is no doubt that strategies such as progressive relaxation can result in decreased physical tension in certain muscle groups. And, although tension by itself does not cause stuttering, there is also no doubt that a person who is speaking with less physical tension is likely to experience fewer moments of disfluency. Nevertheless, it is not at all clear that a feeling of relaxation in the legs or arms translates to relaxation in the speech muscles. More importantly, it is also not clear that teaching a child progressive relaxation strategies or beginning a therapy session with a period of relaxation actually translates to fluency gains in the child's real world (Bloodstein 1995, Van Riper 1973). Indeed, the benefits of being relaxed are typically lost the minute the child is done with the exercise. He sits back up in his chair, tenses up his muscles to their "normal" level of tension, and continues talking as if nothing had happened without attempting to maintain a feeling of relaxation in his speech musculature. Therefore, we do not teach progressive relaxation or other techniques designed to render the child less physically tense overall. Also, we do not expect the child to learn how to relax his whole body in those situations where he wants to speak more fluently.

Of course, if a child experiences overall feelings of anxiety associated with speech, then we may need to address this, and relaxation exercises may play a role in overall anxiety reduction. For improving fluency, however, we do not rely on a general sense of "relaxation" as a fluency inducer. We use relaxation as a tool designed to help children learn to change the amount of tension in their speech muscles and, ultimately, modify their moments of stuttering.

In sum, relaxation can play an important role in therapy for children who stutter; however, the goal of relaxation exercises is not to get the child to speak more fluently during the exercise. Indeed, a therapy session in which the child speaks fluently because he has become relaxed teaches him relatively little about how to communicate in the real world. In extreme cases, this situation may actually contribute to difficulties with generalization of fluency skills. Rather, by using relaxation as a specific tool to teach children about speech production, physical tension during stuttering, and the modification of stuttering moments, you can actually help children who stutter improve their overall communication using activities that are relatively straightforward and fun.

Becoming a "speech detective"

Earlier, we talked about helping a child increase his self-monitoring skills by examining what happens when he is speaking fluently. It is also important for the child to explore moments of stuttering in the same way. Because he may be uncomfortable thinking about stuttering, he may initially be reluctant to explore the physical sensations and movement associated with moments of disfluency. We can help him approach this type of experience by framing our exercise in terms of "becoming a speech detective."

We often begin the speech detective exercises by intentionally increasing physical tension in our own speech, then making matter-of-fact comments about where we felt the tension. We can turn this exercise into a game by increasing tension in different parts of the speech machine (or in other parts of the body) and then inviting the child to tell us where he thinks our muscles are tight. After the child

> ## Sample Dialogue
>
> Here is a sample dialogue that demonstrates how the "speech detective" activity can be used:
>
> "I am going to try to put some tension in my speech. Watch and we will try to figure out where in my speech machine I am getting tight. Ready?
>
> t-t-t-able
>
> See, I got tight in my tongue…right here….t-t-table.
>
> Now, I'll try it again and you tell me where you think I am getting tight.
>
> b-b-baby
>
> Wow…you are really smart about this!"
>
> After several times, the child can be invited to take a turn.

has developed some comfort with the activity, we can take turns increasing tension and "detecting" each other's tension. (Note: For older children, you can call this activity "Identifying Tension.")

Depending upon the child's age and degree of comfort with stuttering, you can even do this activity by demonstrating tension that directly mimics the child's stuttering. In this way, you can help the child locate the tension in his speech machine through interesting and non-threatening activities. The key is to be creative and fun so the child will learn about stuttering and physical tension without feeling uncomfortable with the fact that he is working on his stuttering.

Therapy Activity: Staying in the block

Talking about stuttering, observing stuttering, and listening to stuttering are all good ways to help children learn about their speech. Another helpful technique can be called "staying in the block." With this activity, the child "catches" a moment of stuttering right in the middle and holds onto it rather than continuing to speak (Guitar 1998; Williams 1971, 1979). The purpose of the activity is to help the child become more aware of what he is doing during moments of stuttering. By holding onto the block, the child gains more time to explore the sensation of physical tension in his muscles. He also gains the opportunity to face his stuttering very directly, and this can help him become desensitized to the physical and emotional reactions that may occur during disfluencies.

While the child is holding onto the block, you can ask questions about what his articulators are doing, where he feels stuck, how long the feeling of being "blocked" really lasts, etc. Questions like these help the child to explore his moments of stuttering in a safe, supportive environment and lays the groundwork for further investigations into his stuttering behaviors.

Initially, children may have difficulty catching the blocks while they are speaking. With practice, however, this activity will help children develop the self-monitoring skills they will need for using speaking strategies, including those designed to improve fluency (e.g., easy starts) or to change moments of stuttering (e.g., easing out). These more advanced strategies (discussed later in this chapter) all require children to be able to *monitor* their speech and make changes as necessary to maintain fluency or reduce the severity of stuttering.

If a child has too much difficulty staying in real blocks, he can begin to practice this technique using "pseudo-stuttering" (pretend, or fake, stuttering). With practice, he will gradually become better at identifying when he is experiencing tension in his speech muscles so he can catch the real blocks as they are happening.

One helpful therapy activity is to play a game with the child to see who can produce real or fake stutters, catch them, and hold onto them (Dell 1993, Murphy 1989). You can award points if the child catches you in a block that was "missed," and the child can learn that exploring stuttering can become fun and rewarding. Remember that for this activity, as well as for all other activities designed to educate the child about stuttering, the purpose is not specifically to increase fluency, but rather to give the child a solid foundation for later development of skills that will enhance his speech production.

Therapy Activity: Tension travels

As we explore stuttering in a safe and supportive environment, we can discover that tension does not always happen in the same place or in just one place at a time. Sometimes tension can begin in our lips and travel to our tongue, our larynx, or other parts of the body. Recognizing that tension travels helps a child locate and modify tension throughout his body.

As with other aspects of treatment, you can use creative detective-type activities to help the child enhance his understanding in a way that is fun and non-threatening. You can use the play activities described above for "staying in the block," and then discuss how the tension begins in one place of the speech machine (e.g., lips) and sometimes travels to other points (e.g., tongue or vocal cords). You can model self-monitoring skills by describing in detail the feelings experienced during your own tense moment of pseudo-stuttering. The child can then follow this model by exploring how his own tension travels during moments of real or fake stuttering, and this will help him develop his self-monitoring skills.

Sample Dialogue

"Let's 'detect' our tension in a really tight moment this time. I'll try one first." (Notice that this activity combines both Speech Detective and Staying in the Block.)

"K---eep.

"Wow! That was a really tight one. When I started feeling tension, I felt my tongue pushing up against the 'roof' of my mouth, way in the back of my mouth. But then when I tried to say the rest of the word, I could feel tension in my vocal cords too. My tension was really traveling to different places in my speech machine.

"Now it's your turn. When you do a tight stutter, feel where your tension starts and then let me know if you feel it travel to any other speech muscles."

Easy Starts are just a start

By this point in therapy, the child has learned much about speaking and stuttering; however, he has not yet learned anything that is specifically designed to help him speak more fluently. You have done a very thorough job of "setting the stage" for success in therapy, but there is much more to do.

Often, clinicians are eager to begin the process of teaching the child techniques that will help him improve his fluency. This may be particularly true if the child has actually become more concerned about his stuttering as his knowledge about stuttering has increased. Thus, you may wish to introduce techniques such as "easy starts" or gentle onsets to help smooth out his speech.

Unfortunately, no strategy is completely fool-proof. Although many techniques can help children improve fluency, no technique can eliminate all moments of stuttering in a child's speech. Even if a child's speech improves dramatically to the point where he exhibits only occasional stuttering moments, we must be sure that those few moments of stuttering do not cause the child undue discomfort. Therefore, *before* we introduce fluency strategies, we want to make sure the child has tools for modifying the moments of stuttering that remain. If he does not have such tools, the child is at a greatly increased risk for a relapse if his discomfort about occasional disfluencies develops into fear about whether his stuttering will increase.

Okay, So I Need to Help Him Change His Stuttering. How Do I Do It?

When children stutter, they typically experience a feeling of physical tension in the muscles used for speech production (including muscles of respiration, phonation, and articulation). The more they struggle with their speech, the more this tension builds up. As the tension builds, children may find it more and more difficult to work their way out of disfluencies they are in, and the likelihood that more stuttering will occur increases dramatically. As shown in the figures below and on the next page, when children learn to manage this physical tension, they can begin to experience a general reduction in the amount of tightness they feel in their speech production mechanism, and this, in turn, will help to reduce the amount of stuttering in their speech.

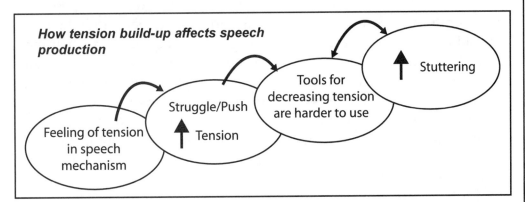

Because of the relationship between tension and stuttering, one of the most important lessons we can teach children who stutter is how to *manage* the physical tension they feel in their speech muscles when they are stuttering. Teaching children strategies for changing stuttering is like creating a "safety net" to help them when their fluency strategies fail, or when they find themselves in situations where it is more difficult to use fluency strategies.

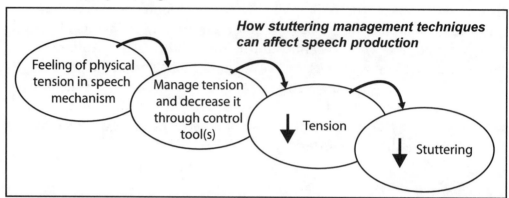

How stuttering management techniques can affect speech production

Traditionally, tools for reducing physical tension during stuttering have been called "stuttering modification" strategies (Williams & Dugan 2002). They are often presented in contrast to so-called "speech modification" strategies, or strategies for improving fluency directly (Bothe 2002). We will address these types of fluency-enhancing strategies in the next section; however, for now, it is important to recognize that we will combine all of these strategies and use both speech modification and stuttering modification techniques to help children achieve improvements in their overall communication (Yaruss & Reardon 2002).

Packing the toolbox: techniques for easier stuttering

For many years, clinicians and people who stutter have relied on stuttering modification techniques such as "cancellation" and "pull out" (Van Riper 1973). These strategies are designed to help people who stutter decrease the amount of tension they experience when speaking. We have found these strategies very beneficial for helping school-age children who stutter manage their stuttering and become more effective communicators (Williams & Dugan 2002). More importantly, we have also found that it is imperative that clinicians and students both be aware of the *rationale* behind each of the stuttering modification techniques. When used properly, these techniques are not just speech strategies designed to help people talk more easily; they are also life strategies that help people develop the tools they need to face new and difficult situations long after therapy has concluded.

Of course, understanding the rationale for therapy is necessary regardless of the specific strategy that is used. To emphasize the importance of the rationale with these techniques, we have developed a series of summary sheets that review the "what, why, and how" of each stuttering modification tool we present in this section, as well as the speech modification tools and communication tools in the following section. The summary sheets are meant as a review of the details of the tools and can be used to help you, the children, their parents, and their teachers understand them. (The summary sheets, all entitled *Communication Tools*, can be found in Appendix 4B on pages 181–190.)

Cancellation

Cancellation is a stuttering modification technique that is used *after* a moment of stuttering has occurred (Van Riper 1973). The technique has three primary purposes.

1. Decreasing Tension: Cancellation helps a child decrease the amount of tension he feels in his muscles *after* a moment of stuttering has occurred and *before* he proceeds onto the next word or utterance. This helps to reduce the likelihood that residual tension will build up and cause additional stuttering in the child's speech.

2. Increasing a Feeling of Control: Cancellation helps a child regain a sense of control over his speech by returning to the word that was stuttered and producing it again with a different degree of tension. By returning to a moment of stuttering and gaining more control over his speech as soon as possible following the disfluency, the child is showing himself that stuttering is no longer in charge. This can be a very empowering feeling and can increase a child's confidence in his communication skills.

3. Desensitization: Cancellation is a highly valuable tool for helping to desensitize a child to his concerns about stuttering. Because the child must go back to the stuttered word after the stutter is already completed, this technique requires that the child directly face his fears about the stuttered word and his concerns about how others might perceive his stuttering. We will say more about desensitization later in this chapter, for desensitization is a very powerful means of reducing the control that stuttering can hold over a child's communication.

The process of using cancellations is relatively straightforward. There are two key components to a successful cancellation. After the child has completed a stuttered word, he first *pauses*. Then he returns to the beginning of the stuttered word and says it again with *modified* physical tension.

The pause is crucial to the success of the cancellation and should not be skimmed over or skipped. The pause provides the child with the opportunity to analyze the moment of stuttering (e.g., type of stuttering, location of physical tension in the speech mechanism, degree of tension) and it gives him the opportunity to *reduce physical tension* in the specific muscles where he is experiencing that tension. At first, the child may find it difficult to analyze the stuttering and release the tension; however, if he has practiced the technique of "staying in the block" described on page 140, and if he has been effective learning about the speech mechanism and the difference between tense and relaxed muscles, he will find this aspect of cancellation easier and more automatic.

After the pause and the reduction of physical tension, the child then produces the stuttered word again in a different way. Note that the goal is not to simply say the word again fluently. The goal is for the child to practice *modifying* the tension in some way, whether it be through the use of an easy start or through the use of an easy stutter. Unless the child changes his speech in an intentional way that involves the modification of tension, he is missing the opportunity to learn how to stutter more easily, and he is missing the opportunity to consciously take control of his speech mechanism. Here are some examples of cancellations:

- "Fffffollow me." *Pause. Release tension.* "Follow me." (Produced with an easy start.)

- "L---et's go." *Pause. Release tension.* "Let's go." (Produced with an easy start.)

- "Fffffollow me." *Pause. Release tension.* "F-f-follow me." (Produced with an easier stutter.)

Again, it is important to recognize that the success of a cancellation is not judged by whether the child speaks fluently after use of the technique. Success is achieved when the child consciously and intentionally modifies tension as he takes control of his speech. It is imperative that the child understands that a successful cancellation requires that he intentionally modifies the tension in his speech, rather than simply repeating the stuttered word fluently and moving on.

We teach children to use cancellations by doing them rather than just talking about them. Like most tools, learning cancellation requires practice and persistence. An added benefit is that each time the child practices a cancellation, he not only gains skill with this tool; he also gains desensitization to stuttering and a sense of greater control over his speech.

Initially, the child may balk at the idea that he will need to go back after he finishes a stuttered word to modify the tension. This is understandable, for the child may feel that he has had a hard enough time getting through the word in the first place and that it will only be harder for him to have to go back to the difficult word again. As he begins to explore cancellations in a supportive setting, perhaps using pseudo-stuttering and with you practicing alongside him, he will begin to recognize the benefits of facing his stuttering and modifying tension, rather than allowing the tension to get out of control.

Pull Out (Slide Out/Easing Out)

Pull out is a stuttering modification technique that is used *during* a moment of stuttering (Van Riper 1973). The primary purpose of the technique is to help children regain control over their speech and reduce the physical tension they are experiencing right in the middle of disfluencies. This allows children to maintain forward movement of their speech without the necessity of stopping and pausing. (Note: We often refer to these as "slide outs" because that is a name that seemed to help one of our young clients understand the procedures. We have also referred to them as "easing out" to provide a contrast with "easing in," which is described on page 149.)

As with cancellations, the procedures involved in using pull outs are relatively straightforward, and are focused on reducing physical tension. There are three steps involved.

- The child must recognize that he is in the middle of a moment of stuttering and "catch" the disfluency, like he did with the "staying in the block" exercise.
- The child must identify the location and degree of the tension and then reduce that tension. (Note: Some children find it helpful to stretch out the sound a little bit when reducing the tension [Murphy 1989].)
- The child can continue on with the rest of the word and resume speaking with less physical tension in his speech muscles and smoother speech.

Note that a child can stay in the middle of his stuttered moments as long as is necessary for him to gain control over the tension during his stuttering. Sometimes, this may take some time, and other times, it happens relatively quickly. Either way, when using this technique, he must learn that when he feels tension in his speech, he should not go on to finish the word until he has identified and modified the tension. In essence, he should not continue talking until he has regained control over his speech. Here are some examples of pull outs:

"R" *Tension.* "rrrrr" *Awareness of tension.* "rr" *Release of tension.* "radio" *No tension.*

"Llllll" *Tension.* "lll" *Awareness of tension.* "lll" *Release of tension.* "look"

Sometimes, when children are experiencing a particularly tense block, they can initiate their pull out with a "bounce" or easy stutter. For example:

"Wwww" *Tension.* "www" *Awareness.* "w- w- release w- we"* (produced with an easy stutter)

In pull outs, the modification is made *during* the disfluency rather than afterward and this is the key benefit of the technique, for it results in more fluent and natural sounding speech. Still, this benefit comes at the cost of greater difficulty and a greater need for practice. Again, as with cancellation, we often introduce pull outs using pseudo-stuttering so the child can practice using various types of disfluencies (e.g., repetitions, prolongations, blocks), and differing degrees of tension (Dell 1993, Murphy 1989). Each time, the child can practice creating tension, staying in the moment while releasing the tension, and then moving on and continuing with the rest of the word.

We also help children understand the process and concepts of pull outs through the use of non-speech analogies. For example, children can practice creating and gradually releasing tension in parts of the body other than the speech muscles (e.g., hands, arms, legs, forehead). In addition to being a fun activity for children, this helps to reinforce the notion that they are in control of the amount of physical tension in their bodies, and that they can manipulate that tension at will. Another analogy that we have found helpful is the visual representation of a slide. This picture, drawn by one of our students, best illustrates this analogy of "sliding out" of a moment of stuttering.

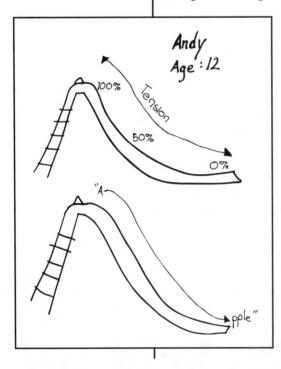

Preparatory Set (Easing In)

The third in Van Riper's set of stuttering modification techniques has been called "preparatory set" (Van Riper 1973). Because this name is somewhat cumbersome for our young clients, we prefer to call this technique "easing in." In essence, easing in is the same as an easy start. Rather than being used at the beginning of a phrase, however, the technique is used at the beginning of a word where the child thinks he is likely to stutter. Thus, the child speaks normally (i.e., without modification) until he feels that he is coming to a word where he will experience tension. Then, rather than beginning the word by tensing his muscles (i.e., using a tense preparatory set), he begins the word using an easy start or other strategy for reducing physical tension. This helps to reduce the tension and increase fluency *before* the moment of stuttering. This technique is most appropriate for children who demonstrate anticipation of stuttered moments as well as the higher skill of being able to recognize this part of their stuttering pattern.

Easing in works together with the other stuttering modification techniques (easing out and cancellation) to provide the child with three opportunities to change the tension in his speech muscles when he experiences a moment of stuttering (Van Riper 1973). Learning these techniques takes practice; however, it helps the child feel a sense of control over his speech and improves his ability to communicate even when he is stuttering.

Variations

In presenting the rationale and procedures for cancellation and pullout, we have highlighted some common variations that children can use to tailor the techniques to their own uses. It is important to recognize that these variations are a critical aspect of the success of individualized therapy. You should never hesitate to work with a child to find different ways of incorporating techniques into therapy. As long as the rationale for the technique is clear, and as long as the fundamental aspects of the technique are intact, you will find a number of ways that children can modify their speech in order to reduce physical tension and increase fluency.

One particularly useful modification that some children may find helpful is really a combination of pull outs and cancellations. Recall that cancellation involves restarting a stuttered word with modified tension after the disfluency is completed, while pull out involves changing the tension during the middle of a disfluency and then continuing on without restarting. A strategy that we sometimes call "block-outs" allows children to halt a moment of stuttering in the middle of the disfluency (like a pull out), then to pause, reduce tension, and restart the word in a different way (like a cancellation). This variation was actually "discovered" by one of our students one day in therapy, though of course we know that many other people who stutter have used similar variations to help them utilize their stuttering modification strategies more successfully in their own speech.

As with cancellations and pull outs, the goal is for the child to reduce physical tension and regain control over his speech, not simply to speak fluently. Thus, when he restarts the word, he can use an easy start or an easy stutter. Here are examples of how block-outs might sound:

- "C-c-c-c" *Pause. Release tension. Restart the word with an easy start.* "Cool"
- "C-c-c-c" *Pause. Release tension. Restart the word with an easy stutter.* "C-cool"

Because block-outs do not require the child to finish the stuttered word like the cancellation does, it loses some of the desensitizing properties of a full cancellation. At the same time, however, it gains some of the properties of the pull out in that it allows the child's speech to sound more natural. Because of this blending of benefits, some children may find the strategy easier to learn. Like all strategies, however, block-outs are not recommended for everybody. Those children who require more work on desensitization should first be taught traditional cancellations, while those children who find pull outs to be relatively easy should focus on them instead. We present block-outs here simply to demonstrate one way that you can work with children to develop strategies and variations that are tailored to their individual needs. We do indeed want children to "make tools their own."

Learning to stutter *differently*

Earlier in this chapter, we talked about how pseudo-stuttering or voluntary stuttering can help children explore the physical tension they feel when they are experiencing blocks. Voluntary stuttering can also be used as a technique to help the child learn to stutter more easily. The technique can involve an easy "bouncing" type of disfluency (Van Riper 1972), a slightly prolonged type of stuttering (Sheehan 1970), or some other modification that helps the individual child. Many people who stutter discover that when they intentionally insert easy moments of stuttering in their speech, this helps them to reduce or minimize the tension that might otherwise lead to harder, more tense instances of stuttering (Dell 1993, Gregory 2003, Guitar 1998, Sheehan 1970). When used in this way, voluntary stuttering can also serve as a tool for helping the child reduce his fear of stuttering in a particular situation. Children can recognize that when they stutter on purpose under their own control, it helps them to reduce the fear of the stuttered moment. We will talk more about the benefits of helping the child become less sensitive or concerned about his speaking difficulties later in the section on desensitization (see pages 170–172).

Aren't we supposed to teach them NOT to stutter?

Of course, the notion that we are supposed to teach children not to stutter is inherent in the idea of speech therapy for stuttering. Parents, teachers, other clinicians, and the general public may believe that our role as clinicians is to teach children to control their stuttering, either so they will ultimately recover from stuttering, or at least so they will no longer demonstrate outward signs of the disorder. In reality, however, our role is to help children learn to manage, cope with, and accept their stuttering so they can become effective communicators. As we have described throughout this book, we work toward these goals through many avenues. Voluntary stuttering is just one of many techniques that can help children move toward a more positive belief system and enhanced communication abilities.

What do you mean "stutter on purpose"?

Sometimes, when we first explain the notion of voluntary stuttering to a child, he may look at us as if we come from another planet. If we want to help him gain the benefits from voluntary stuttering exercises or other strategies designed to minimize the fear of stuttering, we have to make certain that he understands the goals of voluntary stuttering, or "what's in it for him." We need to explain what he can gain from taking the risk and trying some voluntary stuttering. We then need to gradually support him in taking those first steps. We must also explain the rationale behind intentional stuttering to parents, who may need support in accepting that it is a positive thing for their child to stutter on purpose. The discussion sheets on the next page (taken directly from one of our student's speech notebooks) shows how one of our young clients expressed his understanding of the benefits of voluntary stuttering.

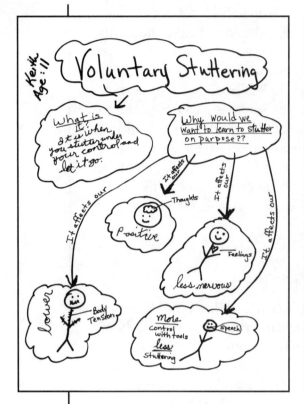

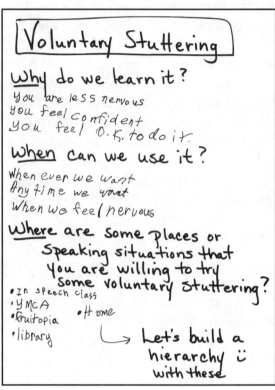

Stuttering—It's not just for stutterers anymore!

It is not easy for children to learn to modify moments of tension in their speech or to try voluntary stuttering. If you wish to help a child learn to accomplish these important goals, you must develop a relationship with the child that is based on credibility and trust. One way you can develop that type of relationship is to show the child that you are willing to try the modifications and strategies right alongside the child.

Thus, if you are helping a child learn easy starts, you must be willing to try easy starts. Similarly, if you are helping a child learn slide-outs or cancellations, then you must be willing to attempt them too. As you move toward strategies such as voluntary stuttering and more advanced aspects of treatment, your willingness to take risks and try therapy techniques with the child becomes even more important. Because most clinicians are not people who stutter, they need to be willing to "put stuttering in their own mouths" through pseudo-stuttering so they can enter real-life situations and practice modifications with the child.

Clinicians who are willing to engage in pseudo-stuttering have a significant advantage over clinicians who are not willing to pseudo-stutter. In addition to developing credibility and trust with their clients, they can also gain greater insights into how to help children manage tension in their speech. By experiencing an approximation of this tension first-hand, they can make more meaningful and more helpful suggestions when they are teaching children to modify tension.

Of course, at first, you may find pseudo-stuttering difficult. Stuttering, whether real or fake, can be embarrassing and uncomfortable. With time and practice, however, you will find that pseudo-stuttering becomes easier—just like your clients do. You might find it helpful to keep a journal of your own as you make your own progress in becoming more comfortable with stuttering. We will say more about the process of becoming comfortable with stuttering in the section on "desensitization" (pages 170–172). Unless you develop the ability to pseudo-stutter without fear or discomfort, you will be unable to help the child in his own attempts to become more comfortable with his stuttering.

Good Places to Stutter

At School		At Home	In the Community
gym	lunch line	with parents	restaurants
cafeteria	bus	with siblings	fast-food outlets
hallway	playground	with neighbors	retail stores
office	classroom	with friends	the mall
library	computer lab		

On the Phone
with people you know
with strangers

How Can I Help Him Speak More Fluently?

Thus far, we have focused our attention primarily on strategies designed to help the child manage his moments of stuttering more effectively. Strategies such as cancellation, block-outs, slide-outs (or easing out), preparatory sets, and pseudo-stuttering can reduce physical tension, reduce sensitivity, and improve the child's overall attitudes toward communication. They can also help the child improve his fluency by reducing the number of compensatory strategies he tries that actually end up disrupting his speech (e.g., speaking with increased physical tension, speaking more quickly or more slowly to avoid blocks).

Our therapy is not complete, however. Though the child may gain some fluency through stuttering modification approaches, we have not yet addressed his fluency directly, and, of course, improved fluency is one of the central goals of therapy for children who stutter.

More tools for the toolbox: techniques for easier speech

There are a number of techniques that can be used to help children who stutter speak more fluently. You are probably accustomed to hearing about different fluency strategies, with various clinicians touting the benefits of one technique or the other for helping children improve their fluency. While we cannot review all of the techniques that have been presented in the stuttering literature, we can focus on a few common techniques that we keep in our "toolbox" of strategies for helping children speak more fluently.

Easy Starts

Easy start, also called *easy beginning* or *easy onset*, is a technique that is familiar to many clinicians. The primary goal of this technique is to help the child minimize the physical tension that may lead to increased stuttering. In essence, this technique involves beginning a word, sentence, or phrase "more easily," or with reduced physical tension (Ramig & Bennett 1997). Some clinicians also encourage children to begin their phrases a little slower at the same time in an attempt to enhance the fluency facilitating effect of the easy start (Gregory 2003). Still others introduce a slight stretching of the initial sound (Murphy 1989).

There are a variety of ways children can use easy starts, and you should be flexible in your application of the technique. Some children, particularly those who stutter more severely, may need to use easy starts frequently in their speech. Others may be able to use fewer easy starts while still maintaining fluency. In any event, each child will require a different amount of tension reduction in order to improve fluency, and you can guide children to use just the right amount of modification in their speech so they can improve their fluency while still maintaining a feeling of naturalness in their speech.

You will find that some sounds are easy to do easy starts with while other sounds are harder. When teaching a child to use easy starts, begin gradually and introduce the technique on sounds that are "easier" to begin easily. Examples of easier sounds include nasals, glides, and liquids (e.g., /m, n, w, j, l, r/). Harder sounds include stops (e.g., /p, b, t, d, k, g/) and, for some children, vowels (since they may be initiated with a glottal stop rather than a gentle laryngeal onset). By beginning with easier sounds, you can give children the opportunity to get the *feeling* for easy starts so they will be more successful when they attempt to use the technique with more difficult sounds.

Ideally, through our "speech machine" discussions, the child has already learned about the different classes of speech sounds, the way they are produced, and the parts of the mouth that are used to produce them. This helps the child play an active role in selecting therapy goals and ensures that the child will understand the rationale for the treatment strategy and practice activities. It must be noted, however, that for young children, you do not have to discuss the idea that some sounds are harder to produce than others as this may contribute to a child's fear of certain sounds. Instead, you can just present the sounds in order from easier to more difficult without dwelling on "difficult sounds." (See Appendix 4C, page 191 for a list of the most common sounds in order from easier to harder.)

Keeping in mind the fact that generalization of fluency skills is one of the greatest challenges facing clinicians who work with children who stutter, we prefer to begin our training of easy starts in phrases and short sentences rather than in isolation or in single words. Another benefit for using easier beginnings in phrases is that it facilitates the development of the pausing and phrasing strategy (see pages 159–160). Easy starts used at the beginnings of phrases rather than individual words sound more natural to listeners and are more likely to be tolerated by the child.

Thus, when introducing easy starts, we create simple phrases and short sentences that begin with words starting with easy sounds (e.g., "Meet me there," "Look at this," "What are we doing?"). There is no shortage of short phrases that can be selected, and the complexity of the phrases themselves can be scaled to the child's level of development or skill. (We have provided some examples in the box on the next page.) Rather than relying too much on preselected phrases, however, we prefer to create new sentences for each child we see. To further enhance generalization, we focus the phrases on topics that are relevant to the child's class assignments or on topics of interest to the child (e.g., *Nintendo* is an easy word to practice easy starts on; *Playstation* may not be as easy.) Often we create the phrases right in the therapy session with the child's help. Then we modify and expand our list of practice phrases each session as necessary. Initially, we may introduce these phrases in direct imitation so we can provide a clear model of the correct use of easier beginnings. From there, we move to delayed imitation or turn-taking games, carrier phrases, structured conversation, and, ultimately, spontaneous speech.

As we work our way up this hierarchy reflecting the complexity of the child's response, we introduce increasingly complex sounds reflecting another hierarchy, moving from nasals, glides, and liquids

Sample Phrases and Short Sentences

1.	I am talented	I am talented at many things.
2.	It is cool.	It is cool to learn about people.
3.	I am responsible.	When I am responsible, I am grown-up.
4.	I am in charge.	I am in charge of my own speech.
5.	makes me happy	Learning new things makes me happy.
6.	It is okay.	It is okay to have trouble talking.
7.	about me	There are so many great things about me.
8.	I like to talk.	I like to talk to my friends.
9.	good listener	I am a good listener.
10.	in a hurry	I'm not in a hurry to talk today.

to fricatives, and ultimately to stops and vowels. Note that different children find different sounds to be most difficult, so we need to work with the child to select the order we introduce the sounds to ensure the greatest possible success.

Ultimately, the goal is for the child to learn to use easy starts *when necessary* (i.e., when he wants to improve his fluency). We do not expect or require him to use this technique (or any technique) all the time. Any clinician who tries to use easy starts all the time will find that it is simply too difficult for a child (or any speaker) to use such techniques with 100% consistency. On the other hand, when the technique is used sparingly, it can help a child achieve fluency when he desires without affecting his speech at other times, thereby improving his overall ability to communicate effectively.

Light Contacts

Another familiar technique, and one which is related in some ways to easy starts is *light contact*. With light contact, the child is taught to touch his speech articulators together with less physical tension when speaking. The technique is similar to the gentle laryngeal onsets that may be taught to a child in therapy for a voice disorder, except that it is applied to all parts of the speech machine.

As with easy starts, the goal with light contact is to help the child reduce the overall amount of physical tension he experiences when speaking with the hope that this will reduce the likelihood of stuttering. Teaching light contact is very similar to teaching easy starts except that it may be necessary to introduce the technique in isolation, at the sound level, or at the single-word level. Some children may find light contact to be quite challenging. It is also important to ensure that the child's intelligibility is not reduced when using this technique. Thus, we often need to experiment with the technique to see if it is one that will work for a particular child. (We will say more about this type of experimentation beginning on page 160.)

What about shorter and simpler sentences?

A wealth of evidence suggests that both children who stutter and children who do not stutter are more likely to be disfluent when they use longer, more linguistically complex utterances (See review in Bernstein Ratner 1997). The precise reasons for this fluency facilitating effect are not clear; however, it is clear that children can speak more fluently when they use shorter, simpler utterances.

The finding that children are more fluent on shorter, simpler utterances can be combined with the finding that children's fluency can be increased when they are praised for producing fluent speech (Harris et al. 2002, Lincoln & Harrison 1999). Indeed, there are a number of very prominent treatment approaches that are based on increasing the child's utterance lengths along a hierarchy from shorter, simpler sentences to longer, more complicated sentences while reinforcing the child for speaking fluently (Ingham 1999, Ryan 1974).

There is a considerable amount of data demonstrating that these techniques do indeed improve children's fluency. Less is known about *why* children become more fluent and what other changes they may be making to their speech to achieve this fluency (Riley & Costello Ingham 2000). Therefore, rather than seeing these approaches as separate from the process of focusing on the child's improved communication and increased fluency, we prefer to incorporate the notion of hierarchies of linguistic complexity and utterance length into many aspects of our treatment. Thus, when we are introducing fluency enhancing strategies such as easy starts or stuttering modification strategies such as cancellations, we follow the hierarchy and begin at an easier level for the child.

What About Slow Speech?

Reducing speaking rate is probably the single most common technique used for inducing fluency in speakers who stutter. Some "slow speech" therapies such as "prolonged speech" (reviewed in Ingham 1984, Onslow 1996) involve reducing a speaker's rate so dramatically that they start out using a slowed rate of perhaps one syllable per second or less. These so-called "fluency shaping" therapies then involve the gradual increase (or shaping) of the speaker's rate to the point where he is using a roughly normal speaking rate but still maintaining fluent speech. Even therapy approaches that do not rely upon dramatically slowed speaking rates still focus in some way on the timing of speech (Williams 1971).

Generally, strict fluency-shaping therapies are only used with older adolescents and adults. We do not feel that these types of approaches are typically indicated for younger school-age children who stutter. We hold this opinion because the speaking style that is used in the early stages of fluency-shaping therapy sounds highly unnatural (Ingham & Onslow 1985). Many school-age children may not be willing to practice unnatural sounding speech in the real-world, even with the promise that their speaking rates will ultimately be increased to near-normal levels. This will limit children's success in therapy and with generalization to real-world settings. Furthermore, research has shown that these approaches are often associated with high relapse rates, particularly for individuals who do not continue to practice on a daily basis following the conclusion of treatment (Ingham 1984). Thus, these techniques may not be appropriate for children who may have a harder time committing to the rigorous practice routines that are necessary to maintain fluency gains over the long term.

Nevertheless, there is much we can learn from fluency-shaping therapies. We can see that a speaker's fluency *does* improve when he uses a slower speaking rate. Note that reducing speaking rate in the school-age child differs from the "turtle speech" that is often used with preschoolers (Conture 2001). For a school-age child, we prefer to aim for a rate that is slower than his normal rate, but not so much slower that it sounds unusual to the child. The less natural the speech sounds or feels, the less likely the child will be to use that speaking style in real-world situations.

Fortunately, we have found that dramatic reductions in speaking rate are typically not necessary to help children increase their fluency. Often, slowing the child's rate just a little bit will improve fluency to a certain extent, and the child can learn to slow down as much as is necessary to achieve the desired degree of fluency.

It is important to note that although slower speaking rate is a common strategy for improving fluency, it is generally not our preference to focus the child's attention too much on his rate of speech. Instead, we prefer to help the child recognize that he can speak more fluently if he adjusts his overall *communication rate*, or the rate of flow of information during speech. Communication rate is affected by speaking rate as well as by the amount of "pause time" the child allows himself to formulate what he wants to say (i.e., the number and length of pauses he uses when speaking). Thus, by focusing on a reduced communication rate overall, we can help the child see that he has a variety of options for helping himself adjust the timing of his speech to enhance his fluency.

Pausing and Phrasing

One helpful way of achieving a slower communication rate with school-age children is to focus on *pausing* and *phrasing*. With this approach, the child is taught to insert pauses between words and, most importantly, between phrases. For school-age children, we prefer this to drastic reductions in the rate of articulation because it helps to maintain more natural sounding speech. Thus, instead of s-t-r-e-t-c-h-i-n-g out his speech overall, the child can be taught to produce speech in natural phrases with short pauses inserted at appropriate places between the phrases and at the end of sentences (Conture 2001, Gregory 2003). The pauses should not be very long — one-half to one second is often sufficient — so the child can feel that the overall pace of speech is appropriate, even though it is somewhat slower than he might typically use in conversation.

Often, for children who are old enough to use reading material in therapy, we introduce the strategy of pausing and phrasing through reading. This offers two advantages.

First, when the child is reading, he can focus his attention on the use of the strategy rather than on the topic of his speech. He can stay at this level of reading for practice until he has developed enough comfort with the technique to gradually introduce conversational speech.

Second, we can facilitate generalization if we select reading material from the child's classroom lessons. This also helps us to ensure that we have selected age-appropriate and skill level-appropriate reading materials.

An example of how pausing and phrasing can be used in a reading passage is shown in Appendix 4D, page 192. Note the double slashes inserted into the reading passage in the bottom passage. These indicate places where the child can insert a short pause when using this technique. Of course, it is not necessary for the child to insert a pause in every location where there is a slash; however, the more often the child uses the pausing and phrasing strategy, the more he will notice an improvement in his fluency. You will need to work with the child to help him find a balance between using enough pauses so that his speech is more fluent without using so many pauses that his speech becomes choppy.

For school-age children, it may not always be obvious where pauses should be inserted. Therefore, we like to have the child mark where the pauses should go when practicing this strategy during reading rather than simply using a prepared reading passage with the pauses already marked. With practice, the child will get a better feel for when to pause, how often to pause, and how long to pause. This will help him find that balance between fluency and speech naturalness that increases the likelihood that he will actually use the technique when communicating in the real world.

As the child develops skill with pausing and phrasing, you can enhance the fluency facilitating value of the technique by combining this strategy with the easy starts strategy described on pages 154–156. Thus, he can be taught to change both the timing *and* the tension of speech simultaneously (Conture 2001, Gregory 2003). Because the techniques work together, the combined use of pausing and phrasing and easy starts will help the child achieve success with all the techniques, resulting in increased fluency and improved generalization of speaking skills to other environments.

Which technique should I use?

It is important to recognize that no single technique has been conclusively shown to result in fluency for all children who stutter. Some children gain success with one technique while other children gain success with a different technique. Furthermore, no technique works all the time. Even if a child is using a technique that appears to work for him, he may still continue to exhibit some disfluencies even when he is trying to use the technique. As a result, it is important for you, the child, his parents, and teachers to be realistic in your expectations. Rather than focusing on "100 percent fluent speech," you must seek *improved* fluency through the use of speech techniques. The specific amount of improvement that a child may gain cannot be predicted in advance because every child is different. Still, it is reasonable to expect a child to exhibit notable improvement using a fluency technique, once an appropriate technique is identified for that child.

Timing and Tension

Although we have only reviewed a few strategies for improving speech fluency in this book, it is likely that you have heard of many more. Examples of various techniques that have been discussed over the years include the following:

- continuous phonation
- airflow
- chaining
- prolonged speech
- easy relaxed approach
- easy speech

Some clinicians have told us that they find the vast array of fluency improvement strategies to be overwhelming, for they feel that they cannot possibly learn them all or figure out why one approach should be used over another.

It is helpful, then, to reflect on the fact that there are many similarities between the various approaches that have been developed for helping people who stutter speak more fluently. Regardless of the name of the technique, most fluency techniques focus on changing the *timing* or *tension* in speech production. It is reasonable for fluency strategies to focus on changes in *timing* and *tension*, for these are the aspects of speech production that are disrupted during stuttering. During a block, for example, the child experiences increased physical tension and the sounds take longer to produce than they typically should.

Thus, light contact requires the child to reduce the physical tension in his speech, and slow rate strategies, obviously, require changes in the timing of speech. Easy starts can involve changes in both timing and tension since the child initiates the phrase with reduced physical tension and at a slightly slower rate. Nearly all of the other strategies can be classified as requiring changes in timing or tension or both. When approaching new techniques then, you can consider which factor is being addressed, and this may help reduce confusion about the different strategies that are available for helping people speak more fluently.

Because we do not know which fluency technique is going to be most successful for each individual child we work with, we often begin this part of the treatment process with a little "trial therapy." Just as we may explore different strategies for helping children with articulation disorders, we may explore different techniques for facilitating fluency. This period of exploration is helpful for many reasons.

1. Using speaking strategies will not sound natural to the child at first. Even though the strategies may improve the child's fluency, he may not like the way the techniques feel or sound because they are not what he is accustomed to. By giving him an opportunity to learn about different techniques, *you can help him recognize that improving fluency will require some type of change in his speech.* This realization is crucial for long-term success, for it helps children understand the active role they must play in their treatment.

2. Exploring different strategies gives the child ownership in the therapeutic process and helps him take responsibility for the changes he is going to make.

3. Exploration of different speaking strategies helps the child realize that he has many options for working on his speech. He can learn that if one strategy doesn't work, perhaps another strategy will. This helps to foster a sense of hope that he will be able to make improvements.

When we find a speaking strategy that appears to help a child—and that the child feels comfortable with—the next step is *practice*. Massed practice is always required for developing skill with a fluency strategy. Practice will be easier for the child if he feels good about the outcome (improved fluency) and the technique. Nevertheless, the practice stage of therapy can still be difficult, and it requires dedication and organization from both you and the child. In Chapter 6, where we talk about the challenges of generalization and maintenance, we will focus more on practice and how to help a child incorporate fluency skills into his everyday conversation.

He's Learning to Manage Stuttering, But He Still Can't Communicate!

One of the problematic coping strategies many children who stutter develop is avoidance of speaking situations. Children may be tempted to use avoidance because it prevents them from feeling the shame or embarrassment of stuttering in front of other people. If a child avoids speaking situations, however, he misses the opportunity to engage in key experiences that help him develop social skills for interacting with other people. As a result, we often see children who stutter who have not developed the same pragmatic skills as their peers. As these children move through therapy, and when they begin to communicate more freely, we may realize that they need help with other aspects of social interaction so they can become the most effective communicators they can be.

Basic communication skills

Often, the people in the environment of a child who stutters are so focused on the stuttering that they do not notice that the child also needs help with basic communication skills. When we look at the whole child, however, and when we focus on a goal of successful communication, we can see other areas that can and should be addressed in therapy. Furthermore, children who stutter have reported to us that they can get so lost in the process of just getting their words out that they have difficulty thinking about social or pragmatic skills that come so easily to other children.

Children who stutter may need help with the following skills:

- beginning and ending a conversation
- changing or maintaining a topic
- attending to and understanding nonverbal cues from their listeners
- using the social skills they do possess during times when they are stuttering

Nonverbal cues may be particularly problematic because children who stutter may over-interpret or misinterpret normal and benign listener reactions as signs of impatience, frustration, or annoyance. In other words, children who stutter may project their own fears about stuttering on the listener. This may cause them to believe that the listener is intolerant of stuttering and this serves to increase their fear of stuttering even further. Of course, children who stutter often *do* face impatience and frustration in their listeners, so it can be very difficult for them to accurately and fairly interpret the nonverbal cues they are receiving.

Working on communication skills

Fortunately, as an SLP, you already possess the skills you need to help children develop their social interaction skills. You can incorporate basic elements of language and pragmatic therapy into your comprehensive treatment for children who stutter when appropriate. In this section, we highlight three key issues you may need to address with school-age children who stutter: eye contact, turn-taking, and resisting conversational time pressures. Of course, this is not an exhaustive list of pragmatic skills that children need to develop, and each child will present needs in different areas. Still, these are issues that we address for many of the children we work with. (Summary sheets of these communication tools can be found in Appendix 4B, pages 181–190.)

Eye Contact

Eye contact is one aspect of social interaction that has received a considerable amount of attention among SLPs. The reason for this interest is understandable; many children who stutter, particularly older children and adolescents, may exhibit poor eye contact when talking with other people. Poor eye contact may be taken as a sign that the child is embarrassed or ashamed about his stuttering. As a result, many clinicians have worked with children to help them increase their eye contact, during both fluent and stuttered speech.

Children need to learn that it is important for them to make eye contact with their listeners. Good eye contact can communicate knowledge, confidence, and trust; poor eye contact can communicate nervousness, anxiety, shame, and discomfort. Still, a child also needs to learn that it is not typical for him to *always* maintain eye contact. The goal of working on a child's eye contact is to help him develop age-appropriate and socially-appropriate eye contact. In other words, as a child who stutters, he should exhibit as much eye contact as his peers do.

To help him accomplish this goal, we need to ensure that the child's eye contact is not affected by his feelings about stuttering. Throughout this chapter, we have described various strategies for helping children cope more effectively with their stuttering. One of the many positive consequences of these aspects of the treatment program is that it will become easier for the child to maintain appropriate eye contact, provided that you also help him recognize the importance of eye contact in conversation. This can be accomplished through role plays and other activities where you highlight the value of using appropriate eye contact.

This broad-based approach to improving eye contact is preferable to frequent reminders to "use good eye contact" or "look at people," particularly if the child is not yet ready to do so because of his feelings about stuttering. Ultimately, as the child gains confidence in his speaking ability, and as his overall communication skills improve, better, more appropriate eye contact will be the result.

Waiting your turn

Proper turn-taking on the part of listeners can decrease the number of times a child's speech is interrupted, and this can reduce the time pressure a child may feel when he is trying to speak (Kelly & Conture 1992). It can be difficult for a child to learn to take his time if he feels that listeners are not willing to wait until he is finished speaking before they begin. At the same time, a child who stutters needs to develop a tolerance for being interrupted so his speech will not be overly disrupted if other people do not wait their turn.

A child who stutters must recognize that turn-taking is an issue that affects both speakers and listeners. Sometimes, a child who stutters may have difficulty waiting his turn to speak even though he knows the consequences for his own speech when listeners interrupt him. The child may be so involved in trying to get his words out that he simply begins talking when he feels he can rather than when he is supposed to. Thus, it is helpful for a child who stutters to learn appropriate rules for turn-taking. As the child's confidence in his speaking abilities increases, he will be better able to wait his turn without worrying whether he will be able to get the words out when his turn comes.

Waiting until you're ready

All speakers feel conversational time pressure on occasion. The verbal and nonverbal reaction of listeners, the amount of time available for a conversation, and the natural competition among speakers for talking time can all contribute to a speaker's sense that he needs to hurry up. When speakers feel time pressure, they may make a number of changes in their speech, such as reducing the number or duration of pauses in their speech, increasing their speaking rates, not thinking as carefully about the things they want to say, or just feeling rushed in general. Most of these adjustments actually increase the likelihood that the person will be disfluent. As a result, time pressure can be particularly problematic for people who stutter.

To overcome the stresses associated with increased time pressure, children must learn that it is okay for them to take the time they need even if they believe that the listener wants them to hurry up. In other words, they need to *resist* the time pressure (Gregory 2003). For younger children, you can attempt to reduce time pressures by helping parents and others in the child's environment give him time to speak and by educating them about the importance of proper turn-taking. Still, we cannot eliminate time pressures from every situation in the child's life. As a result, children must learn to tolerate time pressure and to wait until they are ready before trying to speak.

Waiting to talk can be very difficult for a child to practice, for it requires them to essentially ignore the feedback they believe they are receiving from their listeners. You may need to spend extra time to ensure that children understand the rationale for resisting time pressure. The illustrations below and on the next page show figures we have used to help to reinforce the message that resisting time pressure actually helps children communicate more effectively.

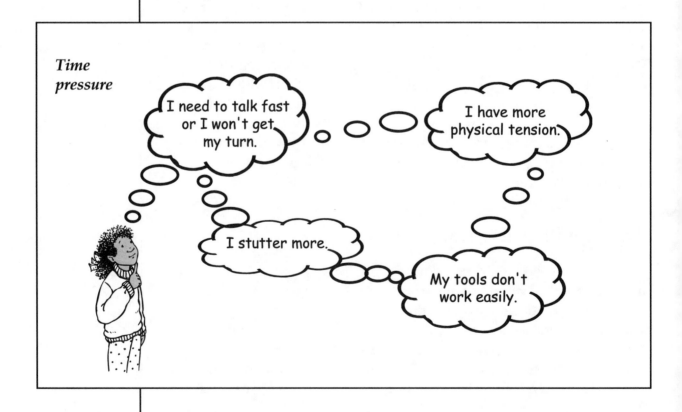

Time pressure

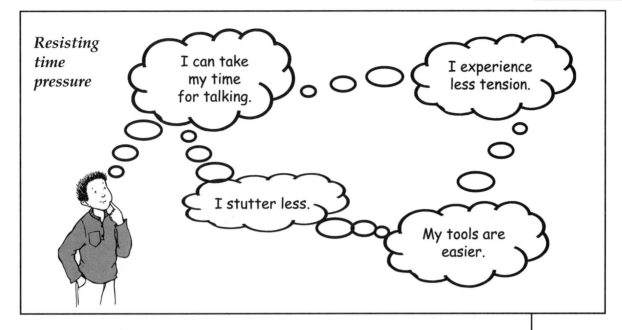

Resisting time pressure

What About that Stuttering Iceberg?

Many clinicians are familiar with the famous analogy that stuttering is like an iceberg with a relatively small proportion of the overall disorder "on the surface" and the larger proportion of the disorder "under the surface" (Sheehan 1970). The analogy is an effective way of highlighting the fact that the observable characteristics of stuttering—the speech disfluencies, physical tension, and struggle—are just a small part of the overall disorder. The factors that cause the biggest negative impact of the stuttering disorder—the child's feelings and reactions to stuttering—are not directly observable, yet we must still incorporate treatment for these intrinsic aspects of the disorder into our treatment if we are to increase the likelihood of long-term success.

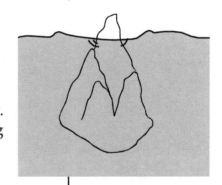

What do you mean "working with feelings?"

Throughout this book, we have talked about the less tangible aspects of stuttering as the *affective* and *cognitive* reactions to stuttering. Affective reactions that can be part of the stuttering iceberg include the following:

- anxiety
- fear
- embarrassment
- shame

- loneliness
- frustration
- depression
- anger

Cognitive reactions may include low self-esteem, a lack of confidence, and the general sense that the child is not good at talking. We can add to this list the behavioral reactions the child may exhibit that include avoidance that prevents the child from participating in key experiences in his life. All of these reactions can affect the child's ability to become an effective communicator; therefore, if we are to be truly successful in helping a child improve his communication abilities, we must address these aspects of stuttering in our broad-based treatment program. We have to help children understand that it is okay that they stutter, that stuttering is not their fault (Murphy 1989), and that they *can* learn to change their speech!

Isn't that for the social worker/psychologist/parent to deal with?

Dealing with stuttering can be quite difficult, and sometimes, a child may exhibit fairly strong emotions. Unfortunately, many clinicians are not comfortable with their skills for helping children and their families deal with the emotional aspects of stuttering. As a result, they may wonder if dealing with these aspects of a stuttering disorder is really part of their jobs or if a different professional should be involved.

It is true, of course, that dealing with a child's beliefs and feelings about stuttering requires a certain degree of comfort with counseling skills. Still, it does not require that you become a certified counselor. If you do not feel that you have the skills for addressing these aspects of a child's treatment, you should not try to engage in counseling without seeking additional input, training, and support. In most cases, however, you can obtain the skills necessary to help children who stutter through continuing education programs, self-study, and through listening to and talking with your young students.

In fact, you should take it as your goal to become competent and comfortable helping children who stutter address the affective, behavioral, and cognitive aspects of their disorders, for this is an important part of the scope of practice in our field (Manning 2001). Because we are the professionals who know the most about stuttering, we are the ones who are best equipped to work with children's feelings and reactions to stuttering (Gregory 1995). Fortunately, we have found that the vast majority of SLPs already have many of the skills they need to successfully help children address their reactions to stuttering. You already have the ability to listen (and to listen well), you know how to respond to different situations children may face, and you care about children's overall success in communication. Furthermore, as we discuss below, many of the treatment strategies we have already described are designed to help children minimize their negative reactions to stuttering as they learn to speak more easily and communicate more effectively.

Consultation with other key members of the child's team, such as the social worker or psychologist, can certainly help and you are never alone in developing a child's overall plan for treatment. If a child exhibits concerns that are beyond your skills, then a formal referral to another member of the team can be made. It is not always easy to know where to draw the line and involve other professionals; however, you can follow the guidelines embodied in the ASHA Code of Ethics (ASHA 2003). Specifically, you should not attempt to provide treatment in an area where you are not comfortable or competent. If you continue to follow a child's progress after a referral is made, and continue to learn about how to work with children's affective, behavioral, and cognitive reactions to stuttering, then you can gradually increase your comfort with these important aspects of the stuttering disorder. By doing this, you will improve your overall clinical skills for helping *all* the children with whom you work.

Learning to live with "it"

For the child who experiences emotional reactions to his stuttering, his long-term success ultimately depends upon his ability to learn to live with the fact that he stutters (Sheehan 1975). This does not mean that he will "give up" on improving his fluency. It also does not mean that he needs to love the fact that he stutters. He does, however, need to come to a "truce" with his stuttering so it does not remain an entirely negative aspect of his life. And, the more severely a child stutters, the more important it is that he learns to cope successfully with his stuttering.

Fortunately, many of the strategies for changing the tension involved in stuttering that we discussed earlier in this chapter also serve to help the child learn to live with stuttering. Many times, however, this is not sufficient to completely help the child overcome his concerns about stuttering, and you will need to address affective and cognitive aspects of the stuttering disorder more directly. Throughout this book, we have talked about the importance of accepting stuttering. In this section, we address specific strategies designed to help the child achieve that acceptance.

Desensitization

Desensitization is the process by which people can become less concerned about issues that bother them (Sheehan 1970, Van Riper 1973). The principles underlying desensitization are fairly straightforward, though the application of these principles requires time, support, and sensitivity to the child's individual needs. To facilitate desensitization, you need to help children face the things they fear, first in situations where they can tolerate the discomfort, then gradually moving toward harder and harder situations as their comfort levels increase. For example, many children who stutter need to become desensitized to their concerns about stuttering openly and freely. To do this, you can begin by helping the child stutter more openly and freely in the therapy room. Pseudo-stuttering or voluntary stuttering is an excellent technique to use in this situation for it helps the child practice stuttering in different ways (Dell 1993, Gregory 2003, Murphy 1999, Williams 1971). This will help the child develop greater acceptance of stuttering in that one particular environment. From there, you can move to other settings that are more difficult for the child along a hierarchy of easier to harder situations such as in the therapy room with the door open, out in the hall outside the therapy room, in the therapy room with a friend, in the therapy room with a less familiar listener, in the cafeteria when nobody is there, in the cafeteria with a friend (Campbell 2003, Sisskin 2002). Note that the order of the situations—and the nature of the situations themselves—will differ for each child (Yaruss & Reardon 2003). Ideally, you will work with the child to determine which situations should be addressed, in which order, and at what pace.

Desensitization is also useful for helping children become more comfortable with speech modification strategies. Some clinicians assume that the child will naturally want to use the techniques because they result in increased fluency. Still, we have seen that many children are still reluctant to use the techniques in the real world because the techniques make them sound different from other children. To help children become more comfortable with the techniques, you will need to engage in desensitization activities with the child using the speech fluency techniques in different situations. Note that this will also foster generalization of strategies into real-world settings. We talk more about generalization in Chapter 6 (pages 219–224). An example of some situations when you can help the child practice techniques is depicted on the next page.

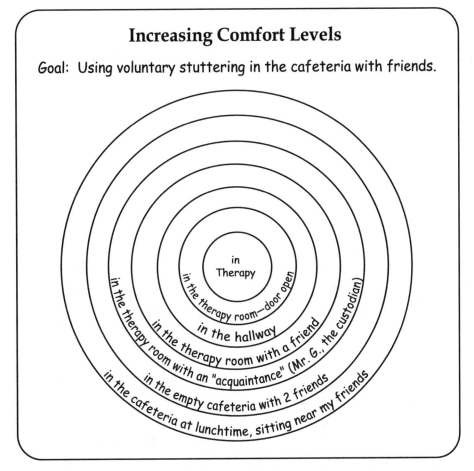

Increasing Comfort Levels

Goal: Using voluntary stuttering in the cafeteria with friends.

in Therapy

in the therapy room—door open

in the hallway

in the therapy room with a friend

in the therapy room with an "acquaintance" (Mr. G., the custodian)

in the empty cafeteria with 2 friends

in the cafeteria at lunchtime, sitting near my friends

Finally, another way to use desensitization and pseudo-stuttering together is to help children "play with their stuttering" so they can explore what would happen if they exhibited a specific type of disfluency in realistic situations (Dell 1993). For example, if the child fears having a long block when talking with a teacher, arrange an opportunity for the child to intentionally produce a long block with a supportive teacher. This will help desensitize the child to his fears about stuttering in front of that teacher. Ultimately, this will improve his ability to communicate with all of his teachers and others as he becomes more able to tolerate his stuttering.

In sum, desensitization is a critical component of the therapeutic process, regardless of whether you are working on goals for improving attitudes, goals for increasing fluency, or goals for reducing physical tension and struggle during moments of stuttering. Desensitization strategies should be incorporated into all aspects of the therapy process through the use of hierarchies that help the child become more comfortable with the goals he is seeking to achieve. By combining all of these aspects of therapy, you will help the child attain his highest level of success, both in therapy and out of therapy.

General techniques for addressing attitudes

For many clinicians, dealing with the affective, behavioral, and cognitive reactions to stuttering can be a challenging component of stuttering therapy. Clinicians appear to "shy away" from this aspect of treatment because of their own discomfort with the disorder, because they are afraid of "making the child worse," or because they are not sure what to say to the child to help him "feel better" about his stuttering.

Let us say at the outset that it is not your job to convince the child that stuttering is okay, or that he should not feel bad about stuttering. The child must come to this understanding on his own. This can be accomplished with your direction and support, but not through your persuasion. Fortunately, many of the therapy activities described above will help children learn to cope more successfully with their stuttering. As children learn to manage stuttering more effectively, the root cause of much of their discomfort is reduced. Furthermore, as they become desensitized to stuttering, their negative reactions will diminish.

Still, there is more that you can do to help children address their attitudes toward stuttering. Most important among these is simply to *listen* to children and provide a setting where they can talk about their experiences with stuttering. Having a stuttering disorder is not fun or easy for children who stutter, but they can benefit greatly from having a trusted, empathetic confidant to share their feelings with. It is our belief that as SLPs, we can play a unique role in helping children who stutter come to terms with their stuttering. Of course, children can and should talk with their parents about stuttering as well, and this is often helpful. Still, if the parents have concerns of their own about their child's speech, or if the parents have not fully accepted the child's stuttering, then it may be difficult for them to be truly "available" to help their child with his own emotional concerns. The same is true with peers or teachers. You, on the other hand, can provide children with a supportive, safe environment where they can come to terms with the fact that they can stutter and realize that they can still do anything they want with their lives. Stuttering does *not* have to be a hindrance to them. They can come to understand this through talking with you, and through their interactions with others who stutter.

Indeed, one of the best ways children who stutter can learn that they are okay is by meeting and interacting with other people who stutter who have overcome their own concerns about stuttering. We will say more in Chapter 7 about how clinicians can partner with support groups to enhance therapy for school-age children who stutter (Reardon & Reeves

2002). For now, however, you should recognize that you are not alone in helping children and families address their negative reactions to stuttering. Through support groups, you can help children minimize their concerns about stuttering and, as a result, improve their ultimate outcome in therapy.

Dealing with embarrassment

Stuttering is embarrassing, plain and simple. As we have mentioned, you can experience this embarrassment for yourself by engaging in some simple pseudo-stuttering in real-world settings. This will give you the opportunity to step inside the world of the person who stutters, even if it is just for a short period of time, to get a sense for what they might experience.

Children who stutter need to learn to deal with this embarrassment. In fact, the more severely they stutter, the more important it is that they learn to handle embarrassment effectively. The desensitization exercises mentioned on pages 133–142 can help children reduce this embarrassment. Talking about stuttering, learning more about stuttering, and educating others about stuttering can also help. As children start to become more open about their stuttering, their embarrassment will diminish. More importantly, as the embarrassment reduces, their desire to avoid stuttering, and the tension and struggle they may engage in to prevent stuttering will also diminish. As a result, the child will stutter with less physical tension, and he will be more likely to communicate more freely and say the things he wants to say, regardless of whether or not he thinks he might stutter.

In addition, learning to deal with embarrassment can help children who stutter in other ways. The child who has learned how to handle embarrassment about stuttering can also handle embarrassment in other aspects of life, such as public speaking, participating in debates or class plays, and approaching new or unfamiliar subjects in school. Thus, children who have achieved success in speech therapy may actually find other benefits in their lives.

Moving toward openness

The more comfortable a child becomes with stuttering, the less likely he will try to hide his stuttering. This is another positive aspect of progress in treatment, for it means that the child will be less likely to engage in maladaptive avoidance behaviors, physical tension and struggle, or other behaviors that reveal feelings of embarrassment or shame. As a child becomes more comfortable with his stuttering, the remaining stuttering moments will be shorter, easier, and less disruptive to communication.

Still, increased comfort with stuttering may also mean that the child's remaining disfluencies will be noticeable to listeners, including peers, teachers, parents, and strangers (Manning 2001). Therefore, as children progress toward the more advanced stages of therapy, they will need to learn how to be open about stuttering. By this, we mean that children will need to be able to allow everybody they speak with to "see" or "hear" their stuttering in some fashion. This does not mean that they will need to talk to everybody they meet *about* their stuttering. It does mean that they need to be comfortable enough with their stuttering that they do not feel the need to hide it—even with unfamiliar listeners who do not already know that they stutter. They may also need to be prepared to explain stuttering briefly, or to acknowledge the fact that their speech is different from that of other people's speech.

As with all aspects of stuttering therapy, this degree of openness can initially be quite difficult for some children to achieve, but it is a goal toward which they can strive. As children who stutter go through their lives they will experience many situations where they need to let the people around them know that they stutter, that they are okay with their stuttering, and that stuttering does not have a negative impact on their lives. This is also an area where we find the interaction with support groups to be particularly useful in helping children achieve enough openness, acceptance, and comfort with stuttering that they can say anything, to any person, at any time, without being concerned about whether or not they will stutter. That, after all, is the ultimate goal of treatment.

Self-disclosure

Perhaps the ultimate achievement, in terms of desensitization, is seen in purposeful *self-disclosure*, or intentionally telling people that you stutter (Murphy 1999, Sheehan 1970). Self-disclosure is an advanced goal that some children may not achieve; however, those who do achieve this goal have truly reached a pinnacle. They have learned strategies for coping with stuttering that will help them throughout their lives and they have learned that there is no reason for them to be embarrassed or ashamed of their speech.

There are many ways you can help the child work toward the point where he will be able to self-disclose about his stuttering. Most basic among these are the activities designed to educate the child about stuttering (e.g., talking about talking, staying in the block, making a speech machine). With all of these activities, there is the implicit requirement that the child acknowledge his stuttering to you and to other children in therapy. The child can take self-disclosure to the next level as he begins to educate his parents and peers about stuttering. (We say more about the value of having children teach their parents about stuttering in Chapter 6, pages 213–214.)

The act of teaching others about stuttering requires, at some level, that the child acknowledge his stuttering. Participation in support groups is another helpful way that the child can continue the process of becoming more comfortable acknowledging his stuttering. Finally, the child can continue using a hierarchy to help him develop his ability to self-disclose the fact that he stutters through specific desensitization activities where he "advertises" or acknowledges his stuttering to key individuals in his environment. He can do this through pseudo-stuttering, distributing educational brochures (such as those available from stuttering support organizations), or interviewing (see box on the next page).

Of course, self-disclosure has to be done in an appropriate way. The fact that the child stutters should not be the first piece of information he shares with new people he meets. And, he should not provide information about stuttering in a forceful way, an apologetic way, or as an excuse for why he cannot do something. Instead, he should simply be able to say, in a matter-of-fact way, and at an appropriate point in the development of a relationship, that he sometimes stutters when he speaks.

The attitude the child conveys when making a statement like this will go a long way toward shaping his listener's attitudes about stuttering. If the child presents stuttering as something to be ashamed of, then the listener may feel sorry for him. If, on the other hand, the child simply presents stuttering as a characteristic of his speech, then the listener, too, will see stuttering as "no big deal" and nothing to be concerned about. In this way, the child can work toward the point where his stuttering truly does not hinder him in any way.

Therapy Activity: Interviews

The interview is a therapy activity that is very useful for helping children achieve openness and desensitization about their stuttering. In essence, the interview requires children to go out into the real world, acknowledge their stuttering, and ask people questions about stuttering. The interview gives them the opportunity to practice self-disclosure, to speak openly and freely about stuttering, to practice acceptance of stuttering, and, of course, to use speech management skills in high-pressure situations (Breitenfeld & Lorenz 2000).

There are several ways a child can do interviews, depending upon the child's particular needs. One of our favorite ways is for the child to develop a short list of questions he would like to ask people about stuttering. Examples include the following:

- "Do you know anybody who stutters?"
- "Do you know how many people in the United States stutter?"
- "What do you think causes stuttering?"
- "Have you ever seen characters who stutter on TV or in the movies?"
- "What treatments for stuttering have you heard about?"

You can work with the child to come up with the questions so he has ownership of the activity. At the same time, keep in mind that the specific questions themselves are not important. The goal is simply to get the child talking about his speech and acknowledging his stuttering to other people.

It can also be helpful for the child to create a brief introduction about the activity so he can explain to his listeners what he is doing. For example, he can say, "I'm conducting a survey as part of speech therapy for my stuttering, and I was wondering if I could ask you three questions." (Notice self-disclosure inherent in the introduction.)

Alternately, you can help the child develop a list of key "facts" about stuttering that he can share with other people (e.g., the answers to the questions listed above or information about how to interact with people who stutter). You can also use literature about stuttering available from stuttering consumer organizations (e.g., "Notes to Listeners" published by the National Stuttering Association or "How to React When Speaking with Someone Who Stutters" from the Stuttering Foundation of America).

In the early stages of this activity, the child may be afraid to approach people and to take the risk of exposing his stuttering. You can help the child to achieve success with this task by accompanying him to the interviews—and doing them yourself as a model—until he feels confident in his ability to talk about stuttering on his own. Furthermore, as with all such activities, we do not take the child out into the real world to conduct interviews until we have helped him achieve a sufficient degree of desensitization about acknowledging his stuttering in easier situations. We also do extensive role playing within the therapy setting so the child will have the opportunity to practice various types of responses that people may have to the exercise. Ultimately, we can go out into the child's community with him, do some interviews ourselves, and support the child as he explores and desensitizes himself to the reactions that he and other people may have to stuttering.

Do children really need to deal with these issues?

Stuttering is a complicated communication disorder that can affect many aspects of a child's life, including educational performance and social interaction. The disorder itself has its roots in linguistic, motoric, and temperamental aspects of a child's development, and the experience of the disorder has affective, behavioral, and cognitive components that can hinder a child's ability to communicate effectively. Because of the broad-based nature of this disorder, stuttering can have a major impact on a child's overall quality of life.

In this book, we have outlined a broad-based approach to treatment that attempts to address all of the complexities of the stuttering disorder that children may experience. Of course, not all children will have needs in every one of these areas, and if a specific child does not have a concern in a particular area, then you do not need to address that area in developing your treatment plan. Still, you must be sure to consider the fact that many children do have needs in some or all of these areas. If you attempt to address only a part of the disorder by focusing only on the observable disfluencies or on the child's reactions to stuttering, then the treatment will be incomplete. This may have significant implications for the child's ability to achieve his goals in therapy and to successfully manage his speech over the long term.

The broad-based approach to treatment is essential for helping children make changes in their lives. This is true of any type of change that a person may wish to make. Before people are willing to make changes, they must do the following:

- believe that the changes are appropriate for them
- understand the rationale for the changes
- believe that they can make the changes (often described as self-efficacy [Manning 2001])
- develop the skills to put the changes in place in their lives

Thus, helping children make changes in their speech behavior necessitates that we also help them make changes in their belief systems (Manning 2001, Shapiro 1999).

Fortunately, there is a large amount of literature from the fields of social work and psychology that you can draw upon to help children deal with issues such as fear, motivation, guilt, shame, self-esteem, and changes in self-talk. We have presented many of these strategies in this chapter. If you adapt these techniques and develop the skills needed to help children deal with these issues, you will see significant improvements in the success of your treatment, and the children will experience significant improvements in the success of their communication.

Summary

In this chapter, we have outlined many different tools and techniques we can use to help school-age children achieve the goal of improved communication. The strategies we have selected include those designed to help children:

- change the way they stutter (e.g., stay in the block, reduce tension, cancellation, easing out, easy stutters)
- increase their fluency (e.g., easy starts, light contact, changes in timing and tension, pausing and phrasing)
- reduce their negative affective, behavioral, and cognitive reactions to stuttering

Throughout this process, we have tried to be mindful of the broad-based nature of the stuttering disorder, the individualized experiences of different children who stutter, and the fact that stuttering is highly variable from situation to situation. By focusing on several overlapping and interacting goals, each of which provides an important piece of the overall puzzle, we are able to help children learn to communicate effectively and participate fully in all aspects of their lives.

"I Can . . . Solve Problems"

Name _____ Grade _____ Date _____

Fill in the blanks with your best thinking and you can come up with your own problem-solving plan. Invite others who may be helpful to complete their own pages.

Name It	The problem is:
Drain Your Brain	Here are ALL the things I can think of to solve this problem.
Look Ahead	Plug in each idea from "Drain Your Brain" and think more about **what might happen** with each one.

I believe if I _____,

then _____.

Group 'em	Decide which ideas are good for you and which may not be so helpful.
	These could work! Oops, maybe not. . .

Pick and Plan	The one I want to try now is:

Rate It	Come back and discuss whether the idea you picked was helpful or not.
	This idea did/did not help because:

Do-overs Allowed!	Go back to the drawing board. Ask yourself:
	• Is the problem listed *really* the problem, or could it be something else?
	• Do I need to brainstorm again?
	• Can others help me brainstorm?
	• Is there something else from my "These could work!" list that I could try?

Communication Tool: Cancellation *(After-the-moment Revision)* —————

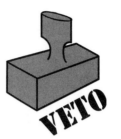

What?   This technique allows a child to take control of the "speech machine" *after* a moment of stuttering has occurred.

Why?   Cancellations help to:

- increase recognition of a moment of stuttering

- create an opportunity for "regaining control"

- decrease feeling that stuttering has won

- decrease avoidance of stuttering

- increase confidence in being able to control speech

- improve communication by increasing the clarity of the child's messages during a conversation

How?   After a stuttered word has been produced,

- pause long enough to analyze the stuttered moment

- release tension in speech musculature

- say the word again using an easy start or easier stutter

Special Notes

- Many times, simply getting the word out feels good to the child. This can reinforce the stuttering or "tricks" over time. Children can use cancellation to minimize the chance that they will use tricks to get through or avoid moments of stuttering.

- The clinician's model is very important. As with all of the tools, clinicians must be willing to provide a model of pausing, then repeating the stuttered word, and practicing along with the child.

- This tool can lead to a positive feeling of not letting stuttering "win" even after it has happened.

- If, when practicing cancellations, the stuttering "turns real" on the second attempt, the child should stay with the cancellation or choose another speech tool until he can say the word again with less tension.

- Remember that the goal is not simply that the word be produced fluently the second time; the goal is that the child modify the tension in some way.

Communication Tool: Pull Out (Slide Out/Easing Out) ——————

In-the-moment Revision

What?   This technique increases the feeling of control and reduces physical tension *during* a moment of stuttering.

Why?   Pull outs can help the child:

- increase the feeling of control

- decrease the feeling that stuttering "wins"

- decrease avoidance of stuttering moments

- create a choice of how to change the way he stutters

- create the concept that he can make the involuntary into voluntary

- continue the forward flow of speech

How?   During a moment of stuttering:

- identify the location of physical tension in the speech production system

- reduce that physical tension while in the middle of the stuttered word

- continue speaking with reduced physical tension

Special Notes

Clinicians can introduce this technique first in a "catching the stuttering moments" activity.

- First, the clinician demonstrates the process of "holding onto the tension" or "staying in the block."

- Next, the clinician can identify the location of the physical tension in the speech musculature, then reduce it.

- Finally, the clinician can gradually continue speaking with less tension.

The child can also practice beginning with voluntary stuttering until he feels a sense of control over the physical tension. As the feeling of control increases, the child and clinician attempt pull outs in sentences with increasing length and complexity, or with higher levels of physical tension.

The clinician can also guide the child to evaluate what is happening in the speech mechanism to help him develop self-monitoring skills. For example, the clinician can ask:

> "How did that one feel to you? Did you ease out of *all* the tension?"
> "On my turn, I felt like I only eased to about 30%. I want to try that one again to see if I can get all the way relaxed . . . ."

Communication Tool: "Block-Outs" *(Combination of Pull Out plus Cancellation)*

What?   This tool helps to increase control and decrease tension during a moment of stuttering.

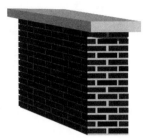

Why?   Block-outs help to:

- increase recognition of the moment of stuttering

- decrease the feeling of being "out of control"

- create an opportunity to regain control

- decrease the tendency to "push through" a moment of stuttering

- decrease the avoidance of stuttering

- increase confidence of being able to manage speech

How?
- identify a "stuck" or tense moment

- stop speaking *in* the moment

- pause long enough to analyze where the tension is, then release the tension in the part of the speech machine that is tight

- continue speaking with an easy start or easier stutter

Special Notes

- It is important to differentiate this tool from simply "stop and start over"!! It is NOT "repeating the word."

- A block-out has many elements that move a child toward *doing something different* with his speech machine during moments of stuttering.

- Emphasize the fact that he is taking control of his own speech and encourage him to be proactive in managing his speech.

- If stuttering "turns real" again, have the child stay with the block-out until he can say the word again with less physical tension.

Appendix 4B, continued   183
The Source for School-Age Stuttering

Communication Tool: Voluntary Stuttering ("Pseudo-stuttering")

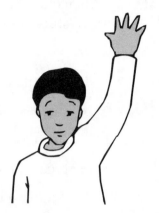

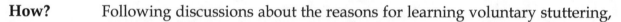

What?   Stuttering on purpose in a *controlled* manner

Why?   The purpose of voluntary stuttering is to:

- decrease fear
- decrease involuntary tension
- decrease avoidance of stuttering
- desensitize to the moment of stuttering
- gain comfort doing the thing he fears most
- increase his ability to be open about stuttering

How?   Following discussions about the reasons for learning voluntary stuttering,

- the clinician models purposeful "easy stutters" during structured conversation
- the child and SLP take turns putting moments of easy voluntary stuttering into speech during structured activities
- ultimately, voluntary stuttering is systematically transferred to less structured settings through hierarchies

Special Notes

- Clinicians must provide a model of acceptance during voluntary stuttering to help children learn that it is okay to take their own speech "risks."
- Voluntary stuttering is a very powerful technique for helping children reduce their attempts to hide stuttering.
- Children may need to *first* feel a sense of control over their speech before they are ready to try voluntary stuttering in conversation.

Communication Tool: Easy Starts

What?   Starting words and sentences with less physical tension and a slightly slowed rate of speech

Why?   Easy starts can help children:

- decrease tension in their speech muscles

- increase their sense of control over their speech mechanisms when they are beginning to speak

- exhibit smoother transitions between words and phrases

- indirectly decrease their rates of speech and the overall rates of communication

How?   Clinicians can model the process of starting words easily, then gradually move into the rest of the phrase.

The child can start with direct imitation, repeating the easy start on the same phrase immediately after the clinician. Gradually, the child can begin to make up his own phrases.

Sample Phrases/Sentences

Say your name.	in the house	over the river
Fix a flat tire.	Land the plane.	Hear a sound.
Make an ice-cream cone.	Think a good thought.	Play the next game.
Wave to your sister.	Be a good friend.	Go to the store.

Communication Tool: Light Contacts

What?   Using softer or lighter contacts between the parts of the mouth used for producing speech (the articulators)

Why?   Light contacts help to:

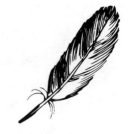

- decrease tension in the muscles of speech production

- develop awareness of the difference between hard or tense movements and light or easy movements during speech

How?   After the child has discussed the parts of the body used for speaking (at a level appropriate for his cognitive level), he can:

- experiment with the concept of *tight* and *loose* or *tense* and *relaxed* in our muscles (Note: This can be done just for the speech muscles or for all muscles in general.)

- discriminate between the physical feelings of tight and relaxed by engaging in play-based activities that allow for the matter-of-fact discovery of how we produce speech

- increase his self-monitoring of the feeling of tension in various speech muscles (e.g., lips, tongue)

Communication Tool: Pausing/Phrasing

What?   When we speak, we naturally group words into phrases. With this technique, children learn to use slightly longer pauses between their phrases.

Why?   Using pause time within sentences helps the child:

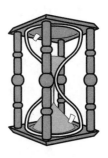

- decrease the rate of communication

- decrease time pressure

- increase the time needed for using modification tools

- decrease tension in speech muscles

How?   Many children need to begin by becoming comfortable with silence. They may need to practice pausing for a second between phrases within utterances. Clinicians may also need to manipulate the situation to "force" the opportunity for a pause. (For example, use sentence strips cut into phrases, place them upside down, and then turn them up as the child says each phrase.)

Gradually, children can practice pausing and phrasing in conversational interactions involving greater time pressures.

Clinicians can model the use of natural conversational pauses between phrases and gradually expand the model to all conversational settings.

When?   The child can learn to use natural pauses between phrases during all conversations. Initially, he will begin with structured phrases, then gradually, he can move to less structured conversation. Note that pausing and phrasing can be used concurrently with all other tools. Thus, the child can combine pausing and phrasing with easy onsets or light articulatory contacts to enhance fluency in conversation.

Communication Tool: Eye Contact

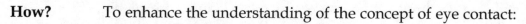

What?   Engaging in appropriate eye contact during conversations

Why?   Eye contact helps to:

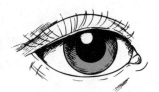

- demonstrate that the speaker is comfortable communicating

- show interest in the listener/speaker

- increase speaker confidence

- let a listener know when the speaker is finished talking

How?   To enhance the understanding of the concept of eye contact:

- brainstorm the positives and negatives of using appropriate eye contact

- during structured activities, use a visual prompt card or signal to guide the child to appropriate eye contact

- integrate the use of appropriate eye contact into less structured situations

Special Notes

- Parents and teachers are not allowed to cue for eye contact in everyday situations. This is a therapy activity only. The child will begin to use appropriate eye contact in conversation as he gains confidence in his communication skills.

- Although we may discuss the concept of eye contact early in therapy, it is a skill that comes with increased confidence *over time*. To decrease the feelings of frustration and "failure," we must not be insistent before a child is ready.

Communication Tool: Turn Taking

What?   Allowing each person in a conversation to feel that they have time to think about what they want to say and to contribute their ideas to a discussion

Why?   When we use good turn-taking skills, we reduce the pressure that may be caused by frequent interruptions. This allows everyone in the conversation to experience:

- decreased time pressure

- increased pause time

- increased time for formulating their thoughts

- increased time to use speech or stuttering modification tools

How?   We develop the concept of turn taking by:

- practicing good turn-taking skills in games and other activities

- talking about turn taking and discovering why it is an important communication skill

- brainstorming the positive and negative aspects of good turn taking

We can further increase the likelihood that good turn taking will occur by providing children with specific language that helps them manage their conversations. Examples include:

> "Are you finished talking?"
> "Sorry Jenny, it's Matt's turn for talking now. Your turn is next."

We can also teach a technique that helps communication partners learn to preface speech in ways that increase turn taking and decrease interruptions, such as:

> "I have a question . . ."
> "Here is something important to hear . . ."

Communication Tool: Resisting Time Pressure (Delayed Response) ————

What?   Using "pause time" prior to commenting or answering a question

Why?   When we understand and use good pause time, we can:

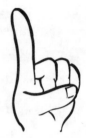

- decrease the rate of communication
- increase time for planning what we want to say
- increase time for using therapy tools
- decrease anxiety about needing to respond
- decrease speech muscular tension

How?   To help children learn to resist time pressure:

- Brainstorm positive and negative consequences of resisting time pressure, for reducing anxiety when speaking, and for improving communication.
- Practice counting to two quietly while preparing to respond.
- Use prompt cards or visual signals during structured tasks to practice pause time.
- Gradually introduce pause time into less structured settings, including those where the child may experience time pressures.

Order for Introducing Sounds When Teaching Easy Starts

When teaching children to use easy starts, it is often helpful to first introduce the technique with sounds that are easier to begin with an easy start (because they involve continuing airflow or movement), then move on to sounds that are harder to begin with an easy start (because they involve some obstruction or stoppage of airflow). This table lists the most common sounds in order from easier to harder, with two sample phrases showing ways clinicians can help children learn to use the technique. Note that vowels are listed as harder because many children initiate vowels with a glottal stop /ʔ/. Note also that dialect differences may affect the specific words and phrases that are used for practicing different vowels.

Sound Class	Specific Sounds	Sample Phrases *(Note: Be sure to work with the child to create new phrases.)*	
Nasals	m n	Meet me there. Need to know.	Men are working. Nice to meet you.
Glides	w j ("y")	What should we do? Yellow is a color.	Where did he go? Yes, it is.
Liquids	l r	Look at this. Ready or not	Let's go. Read the book.
Fricatives	f v	Find the book. Vegetables are good.	Fix the tire. voice is on
	θ ("voiceless th") ð ("voiced th")	Thanks for coming. This is a test.	Think about it. Then we will
	s z ʃ ("sh")	Say you can. Zoos are fun. She will go.	See what we do. Zip it up. Shine your shoes.
Stops	p b	Put that away. Baseball is cool.	Pie is tasty. Buy a ticket.
	t d	Time to go. Don't do it.	Today is Friday. Dinner is ready.
	k g	Kites are fun. Go to school.	Cats are soft. Get some sleep.
Vowels	i ɪ e ɛ æ ɑ ɔ o ʊ/U ʌ	Eat some food. Aces are high. Apples are hard. Oranges are juicy. *Oops* is a word.	in the house Eggs are fragile. Autumn is here. Open the door. up the street

The Source for School-Age Stuttering

Sample Reading Passage
(100 words)

Once upon a time, there was a dinosaur named Hubert. Hubert was a Tyrannosaurus Rex, the scariest kind of dinosaur in the forest. But, Hubert was different. He wasn't scary at all. Hubert liked to make friends and play games with all the other dinosaurs. One day, Hubert was walking through the forest (boom, boom, boom) when he met two little girls! Hubert was very surprised because he had never seen humans before. He thought to himself, "What kind of dinosaur is that?" He decided to go over and say hello, to see if he could make some new friends.

Sample Reading Passage Divided into Phrases
(100 words, 22 phrases)

(Note: Children may put the phrase breaks in different places. Knowing where to put phrase breaks is part of the skill of using Easy Starts and Pausing/Phrasing that comes with practice.)

Once upon a time // there was a dinosaur // named Hubert // Hubert was a Tyrannosaurus Rex, // the scariest kind of dinosaur // in the forest // But Hubert was different. // He wasn't scary at all. // Hubert liked to make friends // and play games // with all the other dinosaurs. // One day // Hubert was walking through the forest // (boom, boom, boom) // when he met two little girls. // Hubert was very surprised // because he had never seen humans before. // He thought to himself // "What kind of dinosaur is that?" // He decided to go over // and say hello // to see if he could make some new friends.

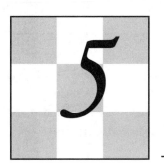

Bringing It All Together

At first glance, it may seem that all of the tools and strategies described in the previous chapter are too much for any one child to learn, or for any clinician to manage effectively. You may wonder whether any child, regardless of her age, can learn to change moments of stuttering through tension reduction strategies, increase fluency through speech modifications, improve her communication attitudes and minimize her negative reactions to stuttering, respond appropriately to environmental reactions to her stuttering, and enhance overall communication success by focusing on pragmatic skills.

To be sure, comprehensive therapy for children who stutter can be a tall order. Still, there are a number of factors you should keep in mind when considering the scope of treatment for children who stutter. First, all children are different, and not all children will require all of these components of therapy. While some school-age children who stutter will definitely need to work on their communication attitudes and become desensitized to stuttering, others will not. Those children who do not need to work on communication attitudes and desensitization can focus more directly on fluency skills. Second, although we have presented goals for improving attitudes separately from goals for modifying stuttering, and goals for modifying stuttering separately from goals for improving fluency, in actuality, these various components of therapy all interact with one another. This helps the child achieve progress on several fronts simultaneously. As a child learns about stuttering and practices modifying moments of disfluency, she is also becoming desensitized to stuttering. This, in turn, reduces the number of disruptions in her overall speech. Therefore, you should not view stuttering therapy as a long series of independent, mutually exclusive goals, but rather as an integrated whole, with the ultimate aim being improved communication.

How Do I Write Goals for All of This Stuff?

Regardless of your work setting, one of the most fundamental aspects of clinical practice involves developing and writing treatment goals.

Throughout this book, we have talked about the types of goals that are appropriate for school-age children who stutter, and we have emphasized the importance of knowing the rationale for each of these goals in the context of a broad-based understanding of the stuttering disorder.

Adopting a broad-based view of stuttering and a broad-based approach to treatment has significant implications for the types of goals that you will write (Olson & Bohlman 2002, Sisskin 2002). It is imperative that you write goals that reflect the wide range of areas you are addressing in therapy. Unless information about treatment goals for modifying stuttering, reducing tension, improving attitudes, addressing environmental issues, and increasing participation are included, then parents and teachers may persist in the misconception that therapy for stuttering is supposed to focus solely on fluency. Furthermore, unless you measure changes across a variety of domains, then you will not be able to document the outcomes of therapy in all of the areas you have treated.

Clinicians often ask us for a list of the goals that we use in therapy for school-age children who stutter. We always hesitate to provide a set or predetermined list of goals, because every child is different and every child needs different goals. Nevertheless, some examples of goals are listed below that address the broad range of outcomes we attempt to achieve in treatment. Again, it is not sufficient to include goals in just one of these areas; if we wish to help the child with the full impact of her stuttering disorder, then we need to write goals for the child that address all areas affected by the stuttering. In each of the following sections, we have created one sample annual goal and several sample objectives/benchmarks. Of course, these are just suggestions and you can adjust and add to meet the needs of your setting and the needs of the children with whom you work.

Goals for changing fluency

As noted in Chapter 3, aspects of therapy that are aimed at improving the child's speech fluency include strategies for changing timing and tension in speech production.

Sample annual goal:
- The child will demonstrate use of learned fluency strategies in 3 of 4 classroom situations as reported by the child and teacher and documented by checklists and targeted observations.

Sample objectives/benchmarks:

- Child will exhibit the use of easy starts 80% of the time in a structured task (e.g., question and answer game) when cued by the clinician.
- Child will exhibit the use of slowed speaking rate during a reading task without reminder cues from the clinician.
- Child will exhibit the use of appropriate pausing and phrasing for 80% of utterances in spontaneous speech.

Note that these goals do not specify a particular level of fluency. As we have previously stressed, it is critical to realize that the child should not be expected to achieve an arbitrary fluency criterion. There are many reasons for this. Most important is the fact that the child does not actually have control over when she stutters and when she is fluent. Sometimes, children will stutter even if they use a technique appropriately (i.e., they are doing what we trained them to do in therapy), and sometimes they will not stutter even when they forget to use the technique. In reality, the only thing the child really has control over is whether she attempts to use the technique taught in therapy. Thus, avoid goals such as "child will exhibit normal fluency 95% of the time" or "child will produce fewer than 5 disfluencies per 100 words in a conversational sample." The attainment or continuation of this type of goal may have absolutely nothing to do with the child's success in therapy. Since our therapy goal is for the child to learn to use communication techniques, then this is what we should seek to measure.

Still, we do count disfluencies, either to examine whether a particular technique is helpful for a child or because we are forced to by district or payer policies. In these situations, it is important to remember that the criteria for successful outcomes from stuttering therapy are not the same as those from articulation therapy. For a child with articulation concerns, achieving 80% success is often viewed as a sign of success. A child who is 80% fluent, on the other hand, is still exhibiting stuttering on 20% of her words. Depending on the nature of the child's disfluencies, this may represent a moderate to severe stuttering disorder.

Goals for changing stuttering

Aspects of therapy that are aimed at reducing the physical tension during the child's stuttering include goals for learning about the speech production mechanism, exploring the nature of the child's blocks, modifying tension, and reducing fear and sensitivity about stuttering.

Sample annual goal:

- The child will demonstrate the ability to modify physical tension in speech musculature using her own choice of tools during 4 of 5 activities represented on her hierarchy.

Sample objectives/benchmarks:

- Child will exhibit the ability to explain the key components of the speech production mechanism to the clinician when prompted.
- Child will demonstrate the ability to increase or decrease physical tension in various parts of the speech mechanism following the clinician's model.
- Child will exhibit the ability to use the easing out technique 80% of the time without reminder cues from the clinician.

Note that the objectives/benchmarks for changing stuttering do not always involve percentages, making the measurement of treatment outcomes somewhat different from what you might be accustomed to. Still, this does not mean that such objectives are not measurable. We will say more about the measurement and documentation of treatment gains in the next section (see pages 198–200).

Goals for addressing attitudes

Recall that many of the goals for changing stuttering also result in changes to the child's communication attitudes. That is not always enough, however, to address the child's needs in this area. Thus, we may also need to write goals and objectives that are specifically designed to reduce the child's negative affective, behavioral, and cognitive reactions to stuttering.

Sample annual goal:

- The child will actively participate in 5 of 7 activities designed to decrease fear of stuttered moments.

Sample objectives/benchmarks:

- Child will demonstrate the ability to use pseudo-stuttering in a familiar situation when prompted by the clinician.

- Child will demonstrate the ability to educate a peer about stuttering when asked by the peer.
- Child will brainstorm about appropriate responses to teasing and use these responses on at least one occasion during role-play activities in therapy.
- Child will reduce the use of avoidance strategies when reading aloud in class.
- Child will report increased acceptance of stuttering and increased willingness to stutter openly when speaking with familiar listeners.
- Child will demonstrate the ability to stutter openly and freely in spontaneous conversation with unfamiliar listeners.

The attainment of these objectives may be verified both by observation and by the child's self-report. Self-report contributes valuable information to our data collection that we may not be able to gain in other ways (Ingham & Cordes 1997). Still, self-report can only become a valid means of assessing the outcomes of therapy if the child is aware of the goals of treatment and if she fully understands the basis for those goals. We have already emphasized the importance of ensuring that the child is an active participant in her therapy, and self-reported progress documentation is just another example of why it is important to ensure that the child understands the rationale for her therapy.

Goals for reducing the impact of stuttering

Finally, as we look toward the overall impact of stuttering on the child's ability to communicate, we can see that many of the goals that we have written so far are also aimed at reducing the negative impact of stuttering. We can address the impact of stuttering even more directly by focusing on those situations where the child may not be fully participating in educational, social, or vocational opportunities.

Sample annual goal:
- The child will demonstrate attainment and maintenance of effective communication in a variety of settings as measured by checklists, self-reports, and structured observations.

Sample objectives/benchmarks:
- Child will read aloud in class when asked.
- Child will participate in group activities at the level expected by her teacher.
- Child will ask questions or provide answers in class at the level appropriate for her overall performance in class.
- Child will give presentations in class in the manner expected for children her age.

Again, attainment of these goals may need to be verified through the report of the child, or of the teacher and others in the child's environment. All of these goals are focused on making sure that the child is participating at a level that is appropriate for her. There is no arbitrary standard of achievement because all children are different. The overall goal is to ensure that the child is getting as much out of her social, vocational, and educational opportunities as she can.

How Do I Measure That?

You will notice that the sample goals listed above are not always framed in terms of percentages such as "80% of the time." Although you may be familiar with writing goals in this fashion, it is important to recognize that these types of percentages are not actually required by federal legislation (Olson & Bohlman 2002). To be sure, goals must be stated in an objective, measurable fashion; however, this does not mean that goals must be based on success in a set percentage of trials or attempts.

Another way of looking at goals is to develop a list of achievements the child can pursue along a hierarchy from easier situations to harder situations. For example, if the child's goal is for her to be able to educate others about stuttering, it does not make sense to say she should be able to do this "80% of the time" or "with 80% accuracy." Instead, we need to ensure that she can demonstrate the skill in a variety of situations, such as "with the clinician," "with a peer," "with her parents," "with an unfamiliar listener," etc. Measurement of the child's ability to achieve the goal in different situations is easy; if she does it, she gets a "check" indicating success in that situation. If she has not yet done it, then no "check" is recorded.

You, the child, the child's parents, and the child's teachers can see how far the child has come in achieving her goals by counting up the number of "checks" on her goal chart and comparing that to the total number of situations that were outlined in the child's hierarchy. Thus, if a child has achieved a goal such as educating others about stuttering in 7 out of 10 situations on this hierarchy, we can say "70% of her goal is achieved" if a percentage is required by a district or administrator. This approach allows you to measure a child's progress in a flexible fashion that is consistent with the types of goals that are relevant for children who stutter. This type of measurement is also consistent with the documentation requirements of IDEA 1997.

Schools Alert: What does "educationally relevant" really mean?

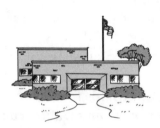

The phrase "educationally relevant" is probably familiar to all school-based clinicians. The phrase comes from the Individuals with Disabilities Education Act (IDEA 1997). Unfortunately, however, the phrase has been interpreted in many ways, most of which do not adequately reflect the intent of the law. In basic terms, "educationally relevant" means that goals must address areas of importance in the academic setting. This does not mean, however, that goals must focus solely on academic issues.

Stuttering can affect a child's success in academic settings in many ways, some of which are directly related to the production of disfluencies and some of which are related more to the child's reactions to stuttering. Recall the example about the child who stutters infrequently but refuses to read aloud in class (low level of observable behaviors but very high educational impact) compared to the child who stutters frequently but reads aloud in class (high level of observable behaviors but less educational impact).

To provide a better definition of "educationally relevant," therefore, we must remember that our overall objective in therapy is to support the child's communication success in the academic setting. This means that we must be sure to address all of the areas that may hinder the child's ability to achieve success. This means that the phrase "educationally relevant" can actually apply to a variety of goals, including those designed for improving communication attitudes, reducing negative reactions to stuttering, educating the people in the child's environment, and minimizing the overall impact of the child's stuttering in many domains. All of this is in addition to goals designed for reducing stuttering in the child's speech, for all of these components are necessary for the child to achieve successful communication in the academic setting.

How Do I Document That?

Documentation of outcomes is another aspect of measurement that requires careful attention. In addition to counts of behaviors (organized either in terms of percentage or checklists in a hierarchy), documentation should involve a portfolio. This portfolio can demonstrate the child's progress through observations by parents, teachers, you, and the child. You can also include worksheets used in therapy as another means for showing the many ways the child can achieve her broad-based goals in stuttering treatment (Chmela & Reardon 2001).

The child's speech notebook provides the best documentation of progress over time. Recall that the notebook has been used by the child to record her own observations about her speech and her progress in therapy. Because it provides a running record of the changes the child has experienced over time, the speech notebook can be a valuable source of evidence for documenting the child's success in treatment. You can ask permission to copy sheets from the notebook for inclusion in your own portfolio of observations about the child's treatment. If the child does not prefer for you to copy those sheets, you can simply record your own observations as you ordinarily would to maintain documentation of your treatment outcomes. You can also create charts with the child in the therapy session that are specifically designed to document her progress.

Above all, you should be sure to recognize that no matter what your work setting, measurement documentation of the child's progress in treatment is *required*, and that goals should be written in a way that facilitates documentation. That means that goals must highlight objective, measurable outcomes that are aimed at helping children achieve success in all of their social, educational, and vocational endeavors.

How Do I Bring It All Together?

The approach to therapy described in this book involves many inter-related goals that are pursued in an interactive fashion. Because of the complexity of this approach, you may benefit from having a guide to help you move through therapy.

One way of thinking about this approach is to keep in mind that we focus our treatment in four primary areas:

a. the child's *speech* (including strategies that both increase fluency and reduce the tension during stuttering)

b. the child's *reactions* to stuttering (including affective, behavioral, and cognitive reactions)

c. the *impact* of stuttering on the child's life (including her ability to communicate effectively in different situations)

d. the potential effect of the child's *environment*, including family members and peers. (We address the child's environment in Chapter 7.)

As noted above, the treatment for these various aspects of the stuttering disorder are actually interrelated. As we move through therapy, however, there will be times we are working more on one aspect than on another. Thus, at one point in therapy, we may find it beneficial to emphasize the child's reactions to stuttering, and later, we may find that we need to emphasize speech management strategies. *This process of working back and forth through the various aspects of treatment allows us to maximize the benefit of therapy for each individual child.* We must rely on our flexibility, problem-solving abilities, and clinical decision-making skills to determine the best course of treatment for each child we work with.

On-going assessment

The needs of children who stutter change during the course of therapy. Not only does their frequency of stuttering change, but the severity of their stuttering moments changes, their reactions to stuttering change, and the difficulties they experience in communicating in everyday situations change. To adequately match our treatment to the child's changing needs, we must continually evaluate "where the child is" and compare that to "where the child needs to be." This does not always need to be accomplished through "formal" or "standardized" measures. Informal observation, teacher and parent reports, and journal activities can be very helpful for keeping therapy on track. Indeed, some of the most valuable information can be gained through simply asking the child how she is doing on her goals, and if the treatment is moving in the direction she wants. The more active a partner the child has been in the development and implementation of treatment goals, the more easily she will be able to answer such questions. Collaborative treatment planning helps the child take ownership over her therapy (Sisskin 2002). This will have many benefits for the child, both in the short term and in the long run.

Hierarchies

Earlier, we mentioned the importance of using hierarchies as a way of structuring therapy. In fact, nearly everything that we do in speech therapy is set up in a hierarchy of some sort. Articulation therapy begins with discrimination then moves to production of target sounds in isolation, in syllables, in whole words, at the phrase level, and so forth. In language therapy, we expand syntax and semantics in a structured step-by-step fashion that is based in developmental theory translated to clinical practice. Stuttering therapy is no different.

Hierarchies are prevalent no matter which specific aspect of a child's treatment goals are being addressed at any given time (Sisskin 2002). If a child is learning strategies to facilitate fluency, then she needs to be able to practice in different settings starting with easier situations (e.g., in the therapy room), moving to harder situations (e.g., in the classroom with the support of the clinician), and ultimately, moving into harder, real-world settings (e.g., in the classroom during oral reading). Likewise, if the child is learning to use voluntary stuttering as a way of desensitizing herself to stuttering, then she needs to introduce the technique first in a comfortable, supportive environment (e.g., the therapy room), then move into harder situations (e.g., the playground or with a peer who understands her goals), and ultimately, move into real-world situations (e.g., talking with her family).

Note that the use of hierarchies enhances the child's chances of success. If she is asked to use a new strategy or try a new technique in a situation that is too hard for her, then she is less likely to succeed and she will not get optimal benefit from her therapy. We can readily envision a child who may be willing to use voluntary stuttering in the therapy room with a clinician she trusts, but who is not yet ready to use that same strategy in her classroom. Similarly, a child may be able to use easy starts in the classroom but not on the playground. Furthermore, the use of structured hierarchies also facilitates generalization, for it helps children bridge the gap between the therapy room (where they first learned the new strategies) to the real world (where they ultimately need to be able to use the strategies).

An important aspect about the development of hierarchies is that you should involve the child in the development and ordering of the list of situations where she will try new skills. What is difficult for one child may not be difficult for another, so you should not make assumptions about the order of the steps in a child's hierarchy. By working with the child on the development of the hierarchy, we can tailor the therapy to the child's specific needs, and we can ensure that the child will play an active role as a partner in therapy. This will give her a greater sense of structure and order as she moves through treatment and enhance her feeling of control over her speech.

Helpful Hint: Using Analogies to Structure Therapy

Often, you can help children and families understand the process of therapy by using analogies. Analogies are useful because they show a child the complexity of therapy in terms she can understand. One of our favorite analogies involves the notion of "taking a journey." This journey does not have a preset endpoint that must be achieved, a preset course that must be followed, or a preset schedule that must be met. Our speech therapy journey may involve many different destinations and take different paths along the way, and it takes a different amount of time for each child to travel.

Of course, this does not mean that we do not have specific goals in mind for the child. We definitely want to work toward goals of improved fluency, decreased tension during stuttering, reduced negative reactions to stuttering, minimized negative impact of the disorder, and increased support and acceptance from the child's environment. During therapy, however, we can use this analogy to help children develop the flexibility they need to meet their individual goals on their own schedules. This will help create a more relaxed therapeutic environment that relieves the pressure on children to achieve a certain arbitrary standard of fluency or degree of acceptance of stuttering within a fixed period of time.

We can also help children understand the therapeutic process by encouraging them to make up their own analogies to describe how they see speech therapy. Many of the lessons children learn in therapy can best be described as "life lessons." Thus, we can relate many of the skills and topics we discuss to the children's real-life experiences. By encouraging children to create analogies based on their own lives and interests, we can begin the process of helping them to "become their own clinician."

Following are some examples of analogies our students have come up with over the years. These all came as a part of thinking about *why we were doing what we were doing* at each stage of treatment.

- *Stuttering is like a spider web. (The more you fight and struggle against it, the more stuck you can get.)*
- *Practicing speech tools is like practicing for a sport.*
- *Speech tension is like a kink in a garden hose.*
- *Slide outs are like an airplane taking off.*
- *Cancellations are like falling off the monkey bars and starting over by doing things differently the second time.*
- *Learning to live with stuttering is like steadily climbing a mountain.*

continued

When a child develops his own analogies, he gains the opportunity to think about his speech in new ways, to use terms that are familiar and accessible to him, and to relate his experiences in speech therapy to experiences in his real life. Ultimately, this will help him achieve greater success in therapy.

In the following example, Brad, age 14, uses a recent indoor rock climbing field trip to demonstrate how what he learned in climbing a wall helped him better understand his own journey of dealing with stuttering in his life. It is a wonderful example of how he used an analogy to relate stuttering to real life.

Lessons I Learned While Rock Climbing

My name is Brad S., and I am a 14-year-old eighth grade student who stutters. Last year I attended a monthly "speech group." I have also been learning to rock climb. In indoor rock climbing, there are two people; one who is climbing while the other is holding the rope that is connected to the ceiling. So if you fall, that person will catch you. The lessons I learned about rock climbing were many, but they also taught me about speech. Here's how they are similar.

You have to learn and then practice. In rock climbing, we had to practice over and over before we could even get on the wall. This is just like in speech, where you have to practice speech tools in order to get better at them.

You have to take on more responsibility. As we paired up for climbing, I remember thinking that I had not expected to be in charge of another person's safety. This meant that I had to be really responsible. This reminded me of how I used to feel about working on speech. I have learned that dealing with stuttering is my responsibility, and I have to accept more and more of it as I get older.

You have to trust the other person. While climbing, I needed to trust that my partner would not drop me. With stuttering, you have to trust listeners, teachers, friends, your speech therapist, and your parents that they will listen to you and say positive messages. You also have to trust yourself to follow through on your goals.

Effective communication is essential. When people are rock climbing, they have to talk to each other for safety. In speech, the most important thing is to get your point across, whether you stutter or not. The message is more important than how you say it.

You have to conquer your fear. When we started up the wall I think we were all afraid at first. But we faced it because we trusted the person hanging onto our rope. I also had trust in my training, and got less afraid by watching others being successful. So I went up and climbed too. When I speak in front of a large group, I get afraid. Fear has a big deal to do with speech. If you don't face it, you will hold yourself back. If you conquer your fear, you will learn to be less afraid each time.

continued

It's okay to make mistakes. One thing is very obvious to me. It's okay to make mistakes. Because if we felt we had to climb perfectly all the time, we were most likely to do worse. If you stutter, it's not the end of the world. If you say it's not okay, you're putting too much pressure on your speech to be perfect, and then if you do make a mistake, you will discourage yourself.

It's okay to get frustrated; eventually you will get it. There were many times while climbing that we got frustrated. Just like in speech, you keep on trying and you are going to "get it" someday. Have faith in yourself.

It's okay if you fall. You catch yourself and start from there. Sometimes on the wall, I would slip and then catch myself. I just started again from where I was. If you stutter, it's okay and you can pick up your message from where you left off.

If you fall all the way down, start over again. When I fell a long way down while climbing, I started from the bottom but knew I had learned the skills I needed to begin again. We have bad spells in our speech sometimes. It's okay. We have learned what to do, and can start again.

Remain calm. I thought of this because one of our speech teachers is afraid of heights. When she got to the top, she was very scared to start down again, and we all talked to her to help her remain calm. In dealing with stuttering, I have had to learn how to deal with fear and to calm myself down when I am nervous so that I can manage my speech better.

When you're facing the edge, have faith in your support. When we got to the top of the wall, we had to stand on a ledge and then lean out to start going down again. We had to really have faith in the person who was supporting us. When I am real anxious and nervous about my speech, I have faith in the people who are behind me and who support me in whatever I do or say.

You just have to find the right rocks. When I was climbing, my partner and I were giving each other advice about which way to go and which rock might be the best one to go to next. In learning to manage my stuttering, I have found that I need to find the things that work for me. I need to use my own best words to express myself, find my best chances or opportunities to talk, and discover which tools work best for me. Other people can guide me, but I have to find my own "right rocks."

I'm Doing All of This, So Why Is She STILL Stuttering?

As we have noted throughout this book, the ultimate outcome of stuttering therapy for school-age stuttering does not necessarily include "normally" fluent speech for all children. Although many children will make significant progress in reducing the number of disfluencies in their speech, many school-age children who stutter will continue to stutter noticeably, even though they are receiving good therapy and making appropriate progress toward their treatment goals. Therefore, you must also consider ways of assessing the outcomes of treatment so you know if you are on the right track, and so children and their parents will know that they are indeed making progress.

What *is* progress?

For the type of therapy we have been describing in this book, progress can be described in many different ways. For a child who stutters severely, progress may be indicated by a reduction in the frequency of stuttering, in the physical tension observed during moments of stuttering, or in the duration of stuttering events. This is the type of progress that most clinicians, parents, teachers, and children will expect to see. That same child, however, will also make progress in other areas. As a result of desensitization activities, she may reduce her avoidance of speaking situations, so she will be more likely to read aloud in class or talk to friends during recess. She may also experience reductions in her feelings of embarrassment, shame, and general discomfort with her speaking abilities. Overall, she may be more satisfied with her life and with her ability to communicate with others.

These types of global, less tangible changes are most notable in children who exhibit few disfluencies on the surface due to their frequent use of avoidance strategies. Paradoxically, progress for these children may also include an *increase* in the frequency of observable speech disfluencies as the child begins to "let the stuttering out" and engage in more speaking situations (Manning 2001). Of course, this increase in disfluencies will only be tolerable if the child has gained more comfort with her speech; however, the increase in participation can only come as the child gains that comfort. Thus, the child may stutter somewhat more, but she will be affected by the stuttering less, and, in the end, she will get more out of her life overall.

How do I know if she's getting better?

Because the nature of improvement in stuttering therapy is not simply the elimination of stuttering, it can be challenging for you, the child, her parents, and her teachers to know if the child is making progress in treatment and if so, how much progress is being made. To determine whether a child is making progress toward her treatment goals, you must collect relevant data that demonstrate the changes the child is experiencing in therapy. As we have already mentioned, this means that on-going assessment procedures must be put in place in each of the areas where the child has therapy goals.

For goals related to speech fluency, this would seem to be relatively straightforward. If the goal is for the child to learn a fluency facilitating technique (e.g., easy starts), then the relevant data would be a count of how often the child is able to use the strategy. Because of the situational variability of stuttering, it is not appropriate to examine

Ask Ourselves: Am I making therapy relevant for this child?

Sometimes, you may want to use standard worksheets to facilitate various exercises with your young clients. The reasons for this are understandable, for you may not feel that you have the time to make individualized materials for all of the children you see. For children who stutter, however, you can actually provide more effective intervention if you avoid using standard "stuttering therapy materials." In order to make treatment meaningful to the child, try to use materials that are directly relevant to the child's current communicative environment. Thus, rather than using standard reading passages when practicing easy starts, you are better off drawing your reading materials from the child's class assignments. In addition to supporting the child's educational lessons, this will help to foster generalization of therapy gains to the child's real world (Yaruss & Reardon 2003). The same is true for selecting conversation topics. Ask the child what topics she talks about the most, what subjects she is addressing in the classroom that could be adapted to the therapy room, or what classroom activities she finds enjoyable or difficult, etc. Other examples include social studies chapters, spelling lists and sentences, upcoming classroom reports, video game characters, and model airplanes. When we make our materials relevant for each individual child, we not only support a child's success in therapy by keeping her motivated and interested in therapy, we also enhance opportunities for transfer and maintenance of positive attitudes and communication skills in the real world.

Another way to make therapy relevant for school-age children who stutter is to select reading materials that are specifically focused on this population. There is a growing selection of books on stuttering that are appropriate for school-age children. Using these materials can help children make progress on addressing their affective and cognitive reactions to stuttering even when they are working more directly on their speech fluency or stuttering modification goals. Examples of these resources include:

- *Sometimes I Just Stutter* (de Geus 2001, Stuttering Foundation of America)
- *Our Voices* (Bradberry & Reardon 1999, National Stuttering Association)
- *Ben Has Something to Say* (Lears 2000, Albert Whitman & Co., available from the National Stuttering Association)

A list of other resources is found in Appendix 2A, pages 45–46.

how often the child uses the technique within the therapy room and then assume that ability would generalize to other settings. Ideally, you will have developed your goals along a hierarchy from easier to harder situations so the child's success in using techniques can be tracked in each of the specific settings defined in her hierarchy.

You should also keep in mind that it is not necessarily helpful to simply keep track of the child's fluency. Of course, improved fluency is one of the key goals of stuttering therapy; however, recall that many times children speak fluently without using any techniques at all. If you count this fluency as part of the child's success of therapy, you may be overestimating the value of the fluency techniques as a way of improving fluency. (We must take into account the fact that other therapy goals for desensitizing the child to stuttering or reducing the severity of individual moments of stuttering also reduce the overall frequency of stuttering.)

To address this possible concern with the validity of the outcomes data that you collect, you should evaluate the frequency of disfluencies in the child's speech as a way of determining whether the selected fluency strategy is indeed helping the child achieve more fluent speech. Then you can examine how often the child uses the target strategy in her speech to see if the strategy is actually useful for her on a daily basis.

As with all types of therapy, you have a responsibility to ensure that the treatment you are using is actually working. By "working" we mean that the child is moving toward meeting the broad-based goals that have been established for her treatment. Thus, whether the goals involve changes in fluency or changes in attitude or both, the child must be on the path to achieving those goals *throughout* the therapy process.

What about "evidence-based practice?"

In recent years, clinicians have begun to hear more and more about the importance of "evidence-based practice," or using published data as a guide for the selection of therapeutic techniques (Power 2002, Yaruss & Quesal 2002). In the field of fluency disorders, this debate has contributed to a long-standing polarization between advocates of different types of therapy approaches (Gregory 1979). Specifically, there is a disagreement between proponents of treatments that focus primarily on fluency and proponents of treatment that focus more broadly on speech fluency *in addition to* other aspects of the stuttering disorder such as the negative emotional reactions and the overall impact of stuttering on the speaker's life. Obviously, you can tell that the approach described in this book is the latter, broad-based approach.

Unfortunately, at present, the stuttering literature contains relatively few controlled research studies demonstrating the efficacy of broad-based therapies using strategies such as desensitization and counseling (Bloodstein 1984, 1995; St. Louis & Westbrook 1987; Yaruss 1998c). In contrast, numerous published studies demonstrate that changing speech patterns do result in increased fluency (See reviews in Bloodstein 1995, Ingham 1984, Onslow 1996).

Some proponents of the fluency-based approaches have suggested that clinicians should limit their treatment only to those approaches that have been described in the research literature, citing the importance of an "evidence-based" or "research-based" approach (Cordes 1998, Power 2002). Certainly, we value the published literature and agree that it is best to select treatments that have been proven to work. Nevertheless, we also recognize that broad-based treatment approaches have been developed for a very specific reason—they have worked with many of the individuals who have participated in them. The lack of published research evidence for these approaches does not mean that they are not effective; it simply means that there is a lack of published research evidence, and more research is desperately needed.

We also believe that there are many different types of data that should be used to validate the treatment approaches that are used with individual speakers (Yaruss & Quesal 2002). The published literature provides one important source of data, but the specific results achieved with an individual client provide another, far more immediate source of data. Thus, we believe that you should select your treatment approaches from among those that appear to be effective for the particular child you are working with. You cannot do this without collecting data about the child's progress in therapy and examining it over time. The data you collect should supplement published research and provide evidence about the efficacy of that specific child's treatment. Without this evidence, you cannot make any claims about whether your treatment is working. With this evidence, you can feel confident that you are helping the child achieve the specific goals you have defined in therapy.

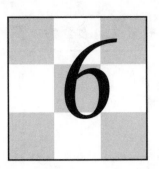

6

It Sounds Good on Paper, but What About in the "Real World"?

Many times, we hear clinicians and parents wonder why a child doesn't maintain his fluency gains once he leaves the therapy room. They can see that he is more fluent when he uses his therapy tools, and everyone wonders why he does not seem to "want" to be just as fluent all the time. There are many reasons for this apparent discrepancy. In this chapter, we will talk about the differences between the therapy room and all the other situations and settings children find themselves.

Why Won't This Child Use His Tools?

Perhaps the most tangible elements of the therapy process we have described thus far are the speech tools—those strategies that are explicitly designed to help the child speak more fluently or stutter more easily. On the surface, one might expect that the child would be thrilled to learn these strategies, for they help to minimize the speaking problem that the child is experiencing. Indeed, it would seem that these strategies should be self-reinforcing. When the child uses easy starts, it is easier for him to speak. Because fluency is ostensibly what everybody wants, the child should be self-reinforced for using the easier beginnings and therefore, use them more often.

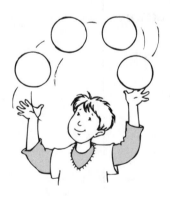

Unfortunately, any clinician who has worked with children who stutter knows that the situation is not so simple. Children who stutter *don't*, as a rule, use their speaking tools consistently. To be sure, they may practice them from time to time, and they may use their techniques in the therapy room. They may even use them in selected situations (e.g., when parents or teachers remind them). Still, it takes a considerable amount of practice and dedication for children to get to the point where they use their tools consistently. This situation may cause concern for you as the clinician, and it can be even more frustrating for the child's parents and teachers. As we gain an increased understanding of the child's experience of the stuttering disorder, however, we will also begin to understand why some children's use of speaking strategies is so sporadic.

If he knows how to be fluent, why doesn't he try harder?

If fluency is so important to children who stutter, why don't they work harder to improve and maintain their fluency? Perhaps the simplest explanation is that using speech modifications, at all times and in all situations, is too hard for many children. Speech is a highly automated task, and making any changes in speech patterns requires a considerable amount of effort and practice. We can see this with children who have articulation concerns. The more severe the child's speech sound disorder (i.e., the more error patterns he exhibits or the more unintelligible his speech is), the more practice he will need in order to improve his speech. Without that consistent practice, he will be unable to make changes in his speech.

What everybody in the child's environment needs to recognize is the fact that stuttering is the normal mode of communication for children who stutter. Of course, it is not normal for other people. Still, for whatever reason, in the absence of intentional modification, the speech mechanisms of children who stutter produce stuttered speech. That is what is natural for the child, and any change from that child's natural mode of speaking will require effort.

There are two consequences to this realization. First, the greater the change that is desired, the greater the effort that will be required of the child. In other words, the more a child needs to modify his speech to improve fluency, the more difficulty he will have doing it. Second, any change from the child's normal mode of communication will necessarily sound different to the child. If the changes sound too different (or, if the child has not been desensitized to his speech modifications), then he will be less likely to want to use them outside of a safe environment such as the therapy room. In therapy, he knows that you understand what he is doing. Outside of therapy, he only knows that his speech sounds different from what other people expect. This may discourage him from using his techniques, even though they help make him sound more fluent. If you keep these consequences in mind when considering a child's progress in therapy, you can begin to recognize the efforts that many children who stutter *are* making. You can also begin to understand why some children seem to make so little progress outside of the therapy room.

Because many children do not consistently try to apply their therapy strategies out in the real world, it is not sufficient to simply teach them techniques and then assume that they will achieve the optimal outcome from their therapy. Solving this problem will require that you specifically guide the child toward learning the value of working on his speech. Indeed, one of the main reasons for a child's apparent lack of effort outside the therapy setting may simply be that the child does not see enough value in the treatment strategies.

Few of us would consistently try to make changes in our speech, or any other behavior, if we did not believe that those changes would truly help us address a problem we are facing. Even though children may know that their treatment strategies help them speak more fluently in the therapy room, they may also know that they have not achieved that same degree of success outside of therapy. An easy start done in the therapy room is far more likely to be successful than an easy start *attempted* in the classroom, particularly in the early stages of learning the technique. That is the time when the child is trying to determine whether the technique is going to be helpful for him, so if he does not achieve success at that time, he will be less likely to continue trying.

If the child is not confident that his easier starts (or any other strategy) will actually help him speak more fluently in the classroom, then he is left with a choice. Either he will simply speak using his normal mode of communication and risk the chance that he will stutter, or he will use a speech strategy that is hard to use, sounds different from what he is accustomed to, and is still likely to result in stuttering. It is not hard to see why many children simply choose not to "try harder." *To help a child overcome this hurdle, you have to help him achieve enough success outside of the therapy room that he will see the value in the treatment strategies.* You also need to help him become comfortable enough with the strategies so he will be willing to use them even in settings where people do not know what the strategies are supposed to sound like.

It seems like he would rather stutter

Parents may become particularly frustrated by the child's apparent unwillingness to consistently use speech tools outside of the therapy setting. We often hear parents ask their children, "Would you rather stutter all your life?" Such statements may reflect the parents' discomfort with the child's stuttering. They also demonstrate the parents' lack of understanding of the stuttering disorder.

As we discussed in Chapter 2, there is no cure for stuttering. School-age children who stutter are likely to continue dealing with their stuttering in some fashion throughout their lives. Thus, no matter whether a child practices and uses his techniques or not, he is still quite likely to "stutter all his life." Of course, the more the child practices, and the more comfort he gains with his tools and with his stuttering, the more success he will achieve in his overall communication. Practice will certainly help, but it is not the only factor that will "make the difference" between chronic stuttering and complete recovery.

When parents begin to understand this fundamental fact, they may at first have to revisit their concerns and feelings about the fact that their child has a chronic speech disorder. Ultimately, however, it will become easier for them to understand and accept their child's sporadic performance in therapy. (Note: This realization and acceptance also take considerable pressure off you, for parents often blame clinicians for the fact that their child continues stuttering even though he is in therapy. In reality, of course, the child will continue to stutter whether he is in therapy or not. The goals of therapy are to help the child stutter less and communicate more effectively, not to convince the child that enough practice will ultimately "cure" him of stuttering.)

This isn't as easy as it looks

Another way of helping parents understand what their child is going through in therapy is to ask children to keep their parents informed about the process. Although this may seem like a simple thing, it is always surprising to us how little parents know about what is going on in therapy. Some of you may use homework sheets, newsletters, or therapy updates to tell parents about their children's progress in therapy. Some of you may not. Even when you do provide this information, it still does not necessarily give the parents enough information about what the child is experiencing.

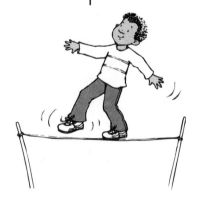

Therefore, we *always* assign children the task of teaching their parents *specifically* what we are working on in therapy. That means that children should teach their parents about the goals of therapy, the broad-based nature of the stuttering disorder, the structure and function of the speech mechanism, the speech fluency strategies, the importance of acceptance, the process of desensitization, the nature of hierarchies, etc. In addition to providing needed education for the parents, this task also helps to reinforce the children's own learning of this crucial information. Thus, we give children this homework assignment *every* session.

Many times, older children may be reluctant to spend time talking with their parents about what they are learning in therapy. However, if they can at least teach their parents about the nature of stuttering and about the techniques they have learned, then parents will recognize when the child is working on his fluency, when he is working on acceptance, and when he is "just talking."

Educating parents about therapy also provides us with one other tool that is very important for those family members who may be over-zealous in encouraging their children to use fluency techniques. Often, when we are faced with a family that refuses to accept a child's stuttered speech, or expects a child to use his fluency technique all the time, we simply require *them* to use the fluency strategies along with the child. We tell them, "rather than *telling* your child to use his techniques, simply *show* him what you want by doing them yourself." The child and his parents can have a friendly competition to see who uses the techniques more frequently.

Typically, there are three key consequences of this exercise.

1. The child does more practice, which is certainly a good thing.
2. Parents begin to recognize that changing speech is not as easy as it looks, and that it takes considerable effort for the child (or themselves) to use strategies.
3. Parents learn to accept differences in their child's speech, and this often reduces the pressure they put on their child to use techniques all the time.

All of these realizations help parents feel less concerned about their child's stuttering, and they ultimately help the child achieve greater success in therapy and in general communication.

Why won't he do his homework?

Even if parents accept the nature of their child's stuttering disorder, and even if they recognize that the changes required of their child are difficult, they may, understandably, still want him to "do his best" while he is in therapy so he can "get the most out of it" and "prepare himself for the future." When parents are evaluating their children's progress in therapy, one of the first issues they may consider is whether the child practices consistently and does all his homework.

You may send the child home with practice assignments designed to improve and transfer his use of speaking techniques. Naturally, you and the child's parents expect the child to complete these assignments, for you know that the child will make better progress in treatment if he practices. In fact, parents who want to be involved in their child's therapy progress may even want to help the child do his homework to make sure he does it. This helps the parents feel better on many levels (e.g., doing the right thing for their child, working to eliminate the troublesome stuttering problem), and it has many other benefits as we described above. Unfortunately, the child does not always welcome the parents' participation. This can add to the parents' concerns about whether the child is working hard enough in therapy.

As clinicians, you know that many children, regardless of the nature of their communication disorders, have difficulty completing homework assignments on a consistent basis. Nevertheless, children who stutter may be particularly likely to avoid doing their homework assignments for many of the same reasons that they do not use their speaking strategies in the real world:

- Speech techniques are hard to do.
- They don't sound or feel natural to the child who stutters.
- They are different from what the child is accustomed to.

Of course, we do not intend to suggest that children who stutter do not need to practice simply because practicing is difficult. They most certainly do need to practice. Still, we do intend to suggest that when you are engaging in problem-solving activities designed to help your young clients get more out of therapy, you should pay particular attention to the reasons that children who stutter may be less likely to practice outside of the therapy setting.

So what are we supposed to do?

Even though we understand the reasons that children may not do their homework, we still want to help them practice as much as possible. Therefore, we believe that you should give children homework assignments, and encourage them to practice. You can increase the likelihood that they will practice by ensuring that they understand the rationale for the practice exercise, and, most importantly, that they recognize the direct benefits of practice. This recognition can be in the form of increased fluency, decreased difficulty in using techniques in the real world, or improved communication attitudes. Regardless of the specific goal you are asking children to work on, it is critical that they see it as worth their time and the considerable amount of effort they may need to expend.

Ask Ourselves: What Messages Am I Sending?

As we discuss practice and motivation in therapy, we can inadvertently send the message "if you just tried harder, you could be more fluent." Indeed, family members may say this to the child directly. As clinicians, this is not the message we want to convey. Telling a child that he could do better if he only practiced harder can increase the child's feelings of guilt about not practicing or increase his feelings of shame and frustration about his ability to achieve therapy goals. There is no situation in which we want to increase a child's or family's feelings of guilt, for guilt is not an effective motivator (Murphy 1999).

To be sure, the child will achieve greater success if he practices more; however, we cannot hold out the promise of success simply to get the child to practice. Instead, we must encourage practice without threatening the child that his lack of practice will have negative consequences and without trying to increase the child's feelings of fear or guilt. Our message to the child must be that *he* is in charge of his speech and that practice can help him manage his speech more successfully. Because he is in charge, he can choose what balance is right for him at different stages in the therapy process. He can also keep in mind that you will be available to help him achieve whatever goal he chooses.

Also, if parents are to be involved in any aspect of home practice activities, two essential guidelines must be set. First, parents are *not* to be involved in practice activities unless they understand the technique being practiced. Second, parents are *never* to take on the role of speech therapist. In other words, they can be listeners and can even be active participants (i.e., taking their own turns in the practice). However, they must be instructed to never correct their child's productions or stop him while he is talking to critique the use of a tool. If they believe that their child is practicing incorrectly, they can contact the SLP to discuss their concerns.

As clinicians, we are the ultimate guides for parents, children, and teachers when dealing with the concept of expansion activities or homework. It is our responsibility to create the optimal atmospheres that allow practice activities to be positive and effective tools for enhancing a child's overall success in therapy.

Finally, as anyone who has been on a diet knows, the more restrictive the diet is, the harder it is to maintain over time. You can apply this principle to the task of helping children achieve success in treatment by simply setting treatment goals and expectations that are both realistic and attainable. "Success breeds success," as the saying goes, and successful use of speech management tools in *some* situations will lead to successful use of speech management tools in *other* situations. By setting goals at an appropriate level (i.e., not 100% use of tools but usage at a level that is attainable for the child), you can help the child achieve greater success in treatment overall.

Encouraging consistency

When seeking to increase a child's practice, carefully consider what you have done to encourage consistency in the child's practice routines. In order for a child to become consistent in his efforts toward change, several concepts must be firmly in place in the child's belief system. First of all, he needs to *know why he is doing what he is doing* in therapy. Second, he needs to know—in very concrete terms—*what's in it for him* if he practices. When a child knows that there is a payoff for his efforts, he can weigh that payoff against the amount of effort it will take to get there. You must make both of these concepts (the rationale for practice and the benefits of practice) clear for every attitude, tool, or situation that is introduced throughout the therapy process.

Strategies that encourage consistency involve:

- guiding children to understand why they are doing what they are doing in therapy
- expanding children's knowledge of "what's in it for them" when introducing activities
- working together with children to set their goals for treatment
- using hierarchies to structure therapy
- teaching children problem-solving strategies they can use when they are facing a roadblock in treatment or in their practice
- developing consistent follow-up or expansion routines (i.e., "home practice") to enhance skills learned in therapy

The *Expansion Activities* form on page 238 (Appendix 6A) can help you and the child develop home practice activities. It is important to note that we try to outline goals for each activity to encourage structure and consistency in practice. We do not, however, set a "determined" number of minutes or person with whom to practice. The child and SLP create the goal, the level of difficulty, and the possibilities for activities. The rest of the details are left to the child and his family. This enhances problem-solving skills, "ownership" in the responsibility process, and an increased generalization of skills to the real-life communication situations of the individual child.

As clinicians, you must also look at your own plans for the child and ask yourself whether your therapy sessions are consistent, whether you actively engage the child in therapy, whether you make therapy relevant and interesting for the child, whether you have a clear goal in mind for treatment, and whether your goals are consistent with the child's own goals for treatment. Asking these types of questions can guide you as you consider ways to help you and the child overcome roadblocks to success.

Gone today, here tomorrow

Be sure to prepare children for the inevitable fluctuations they are going to experience in their abilities to manage their speech. Sometimes, no matter how well or how often a child practices, he is still going to experience significant difficulties in his speech. This can be very discouraging for a child who does not recognize and accept the inherent variability of stuttering. This discouragement may cause the child to "give up" on practice or to believe that more practice (or speech therapy) does not really help.

You can help prevent these negative consequences by actively acknowledging these fluctuations in an open, supportive way without judging that the child has "failed" or criticizing him for not using his techniques well enough. You also need to make sure that the child understands that "what goes down can also come up." In other words, downturns in a child's fluency or management skills do not always mean that the child is experiencing a prolonged relapse.

At the same time, children need to learn that upturns in their fluency do not mean that they are "cured" or that they no longer need to practice or use their techniques. If children recognize that stuttering will come and go, it can help them develop more positive attitudes about the importance of consistent practice and about the long-term nature of success. Children can learn to accept the variability of stuttering as a normal aspect of dealing with stuttering. They can then be encouraged to use problem-solving strategies to guide them toward greater communication success when their speech does not seem to be working the way they want it to. These steps often lead to children becoming more consistent in their practice and more involved in their overall therapeutic process.

Fostering Generalization

One of the most challenging aspects of stuttering therapy for clinicians and children alike is the difficulty that many children who stutter have in *generalizing* treatment gains from the therapy room to the real world. In fact, during a presentation on stuttering therapy for school-age children that we recently gave at an ASHA convention, generalization was cited by audience participants as the single most frustrating aspect of stuttering therapy in a large crowd of practicing clinicians (Reardon & Yaruss 2002).

He's fluent in the therapy room

The fact that children can achieve success with managing speech or positive attitudes on some days and in some settings (e.g., the therapy room), is simply a reality of speech therapy for stuttering that both you and your young students must learn to deal with.

Fortunately, the challenges associated with successful generalization *can* be overcome, and designing therapy with generalization in mind from the very beginning of treatment is one of the most important steps you can take to ensure the success of your clients, both in therapy and outside of therapy, and over the long term (Yaruss & Reardon 2003).

Here, there, and everywhere

The tools we need to achieve success in generalization are largely the same as the tools we need to achieve success in therapy in general. For example, in Chapter 5 (pages 202–205), we talked about the use of hierarchies as the foundation for helping children achieve success in all of the situations they face. By working together to build hierarchies to intentionally and systematically bridge the gap between the therapy room and the child's real world, we can enhance the child's ability to use strategies while at the same time fostering generalization. Similarly, in Chapters 4 and 5, we also talked about the importance of desensitization for helping children approach situations that may be more difficult for them. This is necessary, for all of the goals that are being addressed in therapy, whether they involve fluency strategies, acceptance of stuttering, or education of the people in the child's environment. Again, the use of desensitization not only helps the child achieve success in his therapy goals, it also helps him carry that success out of the therapy room.

To achieve success in generalization, you should seek to ensure that *every* activity is designed with generalization in mind, from the very first session through the very last. Often we find that clinicians wait until the child has achieved a certain level of success in the therapy setting before introducing generalization activities. This follows the traditional model of "establishment, generalization, and maintenance" that is prevalent in many approaches to treatment; however, it ignores the fact that stuttering behaviors are highly affected by the environment the child finds himself in at any given time. A child with an articulation disorder may do just fine if you wait until he achieves 80% success with the production of /s/ in the therapy room before turning your attention to achieving success outside the therapy room. A child who stutters, however, will find this approach to therapy to be detrimental to generalization and long-term success.

Waiting too long before working on generalization prevents the child from developing skills for succeeding in the real world until he is well along in the therapy process. This builds false hopes about the degree of fluency he is able to achieve and sets up inaccurate expectations about the degree of effort he will need to expend in order to achieve success in real-world conversational situations. The child who has not been prepared for the real world from the beginning of therapy will not be prepared to deal with difficult or stressful situations. He (and others) may wonder why he "can't do it anymore" when the same strategies he used successfully in the therapy room no longer seem to work.

Therefore, you should begin to incorporate a wide variety of situations and settings into therapy right away. This will help the child learn that he can modify his speech, reduce physical tension, and accept stuttering "here, there, and everywhere." When you bring hierarchies, desensitization, and the structured organization of the treatment plan together in this way, you can enhance a child's ability to achieve success with speech management skills and positive communication attitudes, to generalize that success to different settings, and to maintain more consistent success over time.

Bringing the clinic into the real world and the real world into the clinic

One helpful way to foster generalization is to incorporate elements from the child's real life into the activities that are used in the therapy room ("bringing the real world into the clinic") and, simultaneously, helping the child carry specific elements from the therapy process out into his everyday communicative situations ("bringing the clinic into the real world").

Talk about the child's world.

To bring the real world into the clinic, you can begin by selecting items from the child's classroom assignments or areas of natural interest (e.g., video games, television programs, popular children's books) to use as therapy materials for *every* activity that is planned. The process of infusing the real world into the therapy can be continued if you invite important people from the child's environment (e.g., peers, siblings, parents) into the therapy sessions. You can always get new ideas about what to talk about in therapy by simply asking children what they are doing, both in and out of school. In addition to fostering generalization for each child we work with, we have found that this provides us with a wealth of information that we can use to make therapy relevant for other children on our caseloads.

Take it on the road.

To bring the clinic into the real world, you can take "field trips" or excursions out of the therapy room where children can practice their skills in a variety of situations that are more like their natural communication settings than the therapy room. Indeed, the most fundamental statement that can be said about this aspect of generalization is this: *to help children generalize their therapy gains to settings outside of the therapy room, you must take children to settings outside of the therapy room.*

To be successful, each field trip must have a clearly defined purpose (e.g., managing fear and anxiety about speaking or stuttering, practicing speech tools with others, desensitization using voluntary stuttering, promoting openness about stuttering through self-disclosure and surveys). In keeping with our general approach to involving the child in all aspects of the therapy planning process, we typically work with the child to select the goals we will work on during a given field trip.

Schools Alert: Getting Stuttering Out of the "Closet"

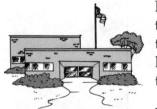 In recent years, a growing number of clinicians have been attempting to take speech therapy out of the therapy room and incorporate it into the classroom. Although this is typically done for children with language concerns, the move toward classroom-based or "push-in" therapy is also a positive development for children who stutter.

The vast majority of a school-age child's communication situations take place in school (6 hours per day, 5 days a week, 180 days per year). Thus, the school setting presents a very real and appropriate setting for generalizing therapy goals into real-life settings. Because school-based clinicians work directly in the school setting, they actually have a significant advantage over clinicians in other settings in terms of helping children achieve generalization.

One way you can immediately begin to facilitate generalization at school is to think of the time spent walking down the halls to and from the speech room as therapy time. During this time, the child can concentrate on a therapy goal while engaging in short conversations with you in a setting outside of the therapy room. This approach can be extended to other settings where the child spends time, such as the lunchroom, the classroom, and the playground. Other examples of generalization activities that can be used in school settings include:

- using materials from the classroom in all practice activities (helps bring the real world into the clinic)

- bringing a friend, a sibling, a parent, or, if possible, a teacher to speech therapy (helps bring the real world into the clinic)

- teaching other people in the child's environment to pseudo-stutter, use easy starts, or modify physical tension (helps bring the clinic into the real world)

- holding therapy sessions on the playground, in the gym, the library, the empty cafeteria, the empty classroom, etc. (helps bring the clinic into the real world)

With the cooperation of parents, teachers, and administrators, you can also arrange field trips outside of the school. You might go to a local support group meeting (especially "youth days" where children and families who stutter can come together to learn about stuttering and provide support for one another). Or, you might arrange weekend meetings of therapy groups at local restaurants or playgrounds. Finally, you can help children use existing classroom field trips as opportunities for practice and generalization outside of the school setting.

You will need to get parents' permission to go on these field trips, of course. Still, the extra effort will help the child improve generalization while keeping practice fun. Together, these factors will help to increase the child's overall participation in therapy.

Private Sector Alert: Stuttering at the Mall

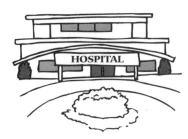

School-age children spend the majority of their time communicating at home or at school. Other settings, such as a clinic, hospital, or private practice therapy room are not as natural for a child, so if you work outside of the school setting, you may have to work harder to help children bridge the gap between your therapy room and their real world. You may need to be more creative in designing and implementing speech therapy field trips to help children achieve generalization.

One activity that we find to be beneficial is to take the child on field trips to stores, restaurants, and businesses in the community. This allows the child to practice skills such as speech modifications and acceptance in a variety of real-world settings while still giving you the opportunity to provide needed support, advice, and feedback about the therapy activities.

Some of our favorite places to visit include:

- department stores (large number of employees and customers to talk to, wide variety of customers)
- grocery stores and pharmacies (opportunity to ask for direction or for obscure items)
- pet stores (interesting questions to ask)
- the public library (other children to talk to)
- the mall (wide variety of people to talk to, opportunities to incorporate time pressure)

You will need to get parents' permission to go on these field trips, of course. Still, the extra effort will help the child improve generalization while keeping practice fun. Together, these factors will help to increase the child's overall participation in therapy.

Once the goal is determined, you can help the child prepare for the excursion by role-playing various situations the child may encounter, including both favorable and critical reactions by listeners. Discuss the feelings the child may experience during the role play, for this will help the child achieve success during the activity.

Most importantly, make the commitment that you will always be willing to take the same risks that the child does during field trips. This means that you, too, must engage in pseudo-stuttering, do surveys, use speech and stuttering modifications, etc. You must also engage in practice and role-playing exercises to prepare for the experience. And finally, you must be willing to share your own feelings and reactions during follow-up discussions. All of this will help you build trust and credibility with each child. It gives you the chance to validate and "normalize" the feelings the child may be experiencing. And, importantly, it provides the opportunity for you to model appropriate reactions to stuttering and successful management of stuttering in real-world situations.

Self-monitoring and self-reinforcements

Another way of enhancing generalization is helping a child develop his own self-monitoring skills (Finn 2003). When a child first learns a new skill, he can rely on you to decide whether he is using the skill in an effective way. This initial dependence must end quickly, however, if the child is going to be able to generalize the skill to less structured situations. Ultimately, he must be able to decide for himself whether he has used the technique well, and he must reinforce himself for accomplishing his goals in therapy.

Any time we explore a new technique or concept, we facilitate the development of self-monitoring skills by asking questions rather than always providing information. For example, when teaching a child to use cancellations, we do not always say "That was good" when he has used a cancellation successfully. Instead, we prefer to ask "How was that?" or "How did that feel?" so he can learn to monitor his own success and provide his own feedback about the effective use of techniques.

It is also important to help children learn to reinforce themselves when they have achieved success. You can do this by highlighting beneficial results of children's attempts to apply what they have learned in therapy. For example, you might say, "When you used that cancellation, you really took control of your own speech." You can further encourage the child to provide self-reinforcement by focusing attention on his emotional reactions when he uses his techniques (e.g., "When you used that cancellation to take control of your speech, how did you feel?"). By linking their actions to positive, desirable outcomes in this way, you can help children learn to reinforce their own behaviors by recognizing the beneficial impact of their efforts to make changes in their speech.

Helping him become his own therapist

Ultimately, the best way to foster generalization and long-term maintenance of fluency skills and attitudinal changes is to help the child develop the tools he will need to independently address problems and roadblocks that may arise throughout his life. Thus, we want the child to be able to:

- evaluate his needs for improving his communication abilities
- identify the outcome he would like to see
- select from among a variety of strategies for meeting those needs and achieving that outcome
- successfully implement the strategies he has chosen

In other words, we want the child to become his own speech therapist.

The tools the child needs to have in order to achieve this goal encompass practically everything we have discussed in this book so far, including:

- observing the current situation (case history and assessment)
- selecting specific strategies for improving speech and reducing stuttering
- addressing beliefs and feelings associated with stuttering
- improving communication attitudes
- using hierarchies and desensitization to help achieve difficult goals
- educating others in the environment and integrating them into therapy
- practicing skills and evaluating the value of that practice
- self-monitoring and self-reinforcement
- creatively solving problems that may arise along the way

All of these concepts, appropriately integrated into therapy, prepare a child to become his own clinician.

Generalization and long-term maintenance can only be achieved when the child learns to ask himself the questions you would ask him, and then use problem-solving strategies to address new situations that may not have been directly addressed in therapy. You can help children develop these skills and then empower them with the confidence necessary to use the skills consistently in a variety of situations. In this way, you can help to create opportunities for children who stutter to become adults who are able to successfully manage their speaking skills, environment, and communication attitudes throughout their lifetimes.

Every Child Is Different. How Do I Adapt Therapy for Different Children?

Throughout this book, we have emphasized the fact that no two children who stutter are exactly the same. Different children have different life experiences and, as a result, require different goals and procedures in therapy. Therefore, you will need to adapt the strategies and plans presented in this book to the needs of the individual children you are working with.

Using age-appropriate language and concepts

When dealing with children who stutter, you will encounter a wide variety of ages, cognitive skills, and levels of awareness. Because of the other children you work with, you have already developed expertise at determining the level of directness or language sophistication a child is capable of handling. Each of the concepts we have outlined in this book can and should be adapted for different ages and varying levels of cognition. As you get to know each specific child you are working with, you can simply ask yourself "What is the most appropriate level to present this information?" and then attempt to adapt the therapy accordingly.

Of course, you will make mistakes. You may initiate a topic at a level that is too simplistic (or too complex), or you may skip a stage of therapy that you feel the child does not need, only to find that the information you skipped would have helped the child with another goal further down the line.

Fortunately, the child himself can help you know when you have hit or missed your target. By observing his verbal and nonverbal behavior, his willingness or unwillingness to participate in therapy activities, his ability to explain therapy procedures and goals to you or to other people, and the overall degree to which he is engaged in the therapy process, you can get a sense for how well the child is reacting to therapy. Of course, this is part of the on-going evaluation and measurement that you must engage in to determine whether therapy is working. This process becomes particularly important when you ask children to take the risks that are involved with coming to terms with their stuttering.

How do you know if he's "getting it"? Ask him!

When you suspect that a child may not understand what you want him to learn in therapy, you may begin to second-guess yourself, asking questions such as, "Is he learning?" "Does he understand anything I am exploring with him?" "Am I doing the right thing?" You may begin to doubt your ability to help the child in therapy, and you may begin to doubt your ability to help children who stutter in general.

When you face these types of doubts, perhaps the best remedy is to simply *ask the child* how things are going in therapy and whether he is understanding the purposes and procedures for the tools he is learning. One of our favorite strategies for gaining this type of information is something that might be called "reflective speaking." With reflective speaking, we prompt a child to explain what he is experiencing in therapy by asking a question such as "so what you just heard me say was . . ." This invites the child to reflect and rephrase what he has heard in his own words. This gives you the opportunity to gauge whether the child has truly understood the concept, and to repair any misunderstandings or misinformation that has been exchanged.

Another way you can determine if a child is following along in therapy is to have him explain the rationale and procedures underlying the skills he is trying to achieve to other people (e.g., peers, siblings, parents, teachers). In addition to helping you assess learning, putting the child in the position of "expert" can help foster a sense of ownership about his therapy and a greater sense of control over his speech (Murphy 1999). It also gives you the opportunity to adjust your course in therapy if necessary. This is just another benefit of working together with the child to create individualized treatment plans, rather than simply involving children in pre-programmed approaches. Ultimately, children who are actively involved in the process of their own therapies have greater opportunities for long-term success.

Schools Alert: But I Have to Group Him!

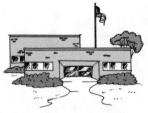

In school settings, large caseloads and time constraints can have a major impact on a clinician's ability to spend one-on-one time with children who stutter. In an ideal world, every child would receive the individual attention he needs; however, this is often difficult to accomplish in the public schools. Still, when we are working on issues such as the difficulty of change, embarrassment about stuttering, and the unpleasant experience of bullying, we find that we need at least *some* private time to help children address these sensitive topics.

When scheduling and caseload restraints require us to group children who stutter, we need to draw upon all of our creativity to identify novel ways to give children individual attention. Here are some examples of how we have handled scheduling for children who stutter.

- Depending upon how many times per week we are seeing a child, we try to reserve at least one session per week as an individual session, and then work with the child in a group for the rest of the sessions. This arrangement allows us to manage larger caseloads without compromising the time needed to develop rapport or to discuss sensitive issues. If we cannot find any individual time at all to work with the child, we at least try to ensure that they are not the only ones in their therapy group who are singled out for discussing attitudes and feelings. If one child has to discuss his feelings about his speech, all of the other children in the group do too.

- When we do group children who stutter, we try to group them with other children who stutter if at all possible. Note that the children in the group do not necessarily have to be the same age; many children who stutter are dealing with similar issues regardless of their ages. Of course, we still need to address those issues in an age-appropriate manner. Still, we often find that such a group can provide a "mini-support group" environment for both older and younger children.

- When we need to resort to heterogeneous groups (i.e., group children who stutter with children exhibiting other speech and language disorders), we try to group children who stutter in language therapy groups. There are two reasons for this.

  1. Much of stuttering therapy is essentially language-based therapy, for we are talking about communicating, conversational interaction, pragmatics and social skills, etc. Of course, there are times when we are also working on specific speech skills. Still, the overall goal is for the child to be able to use these speech skills in the context of conversational interaction.

  2. We prefer to use language groups, rather than articulation groups, because the inherent message of articulation therapy (speak perfectly) may be contradictory to the goals we are trying to achieve for children who stutter.

continued

Thus, a language-based group provides a reasonable "second-best" setting for helping children address the goals of broad-based stuttering therapy, for the message inherent in language therapy (improved communication) is similar to that of stuttering therapy.

At the same time, we know that many children who stutter may also exhibit speech sound (articulation) problems. Therefore, we sometimes find that we can actually create a group of children exhibiting both stuttering and speech sound disorders (Conture et al. 1993). This is generally more likely to be true for younger children; still, as we consider the groups we must create with our young children who stutter, we try to keep this possibility in mind as well.

He doesn't want me to take him out of class.

Many times, the issue of scheduling therapy can be complicated by the fact that the child does not wish to be taken out of class. This may simply be due to the fact that he does not want to miss an important class or activity. Other times, however, the children we work with may not want to be identified as "different" from their friends or as "kids who need help." This is understandable, given the stigma of stuttering and the fact that many children who stutter already feel embarrassment or shame about their speaking difficulties. Overcoming the child's objections requires compassion, creativity, and a clear understanding of the goals of therapy. (Note that the same is true for all children with communication disorders, not just those who stutter.)

First, you need to acknowledge and validate the child's feelings. Being different from one's friends can be difficult for everybody, not just children who stutter. Still, the child's reluctance to admit and acknowledge stuttering will ultimately prove to be a barrier to further progress in therapy, for openness about stuttering is a key aspect of progress. You should help the child understand that developing comfort with acknowledging stuttering will make it easier for him to attend therapy sessions. It will also help him make quicker and better progress in the therapy itself. Accomplishing this goal will require the use of all of the strategies described so far in this book, including:

- implementing techniques to improve fluency and reduce physical tension during stuttering so the child can feel more "normal" and communicate more freely
- desensitizing the child to stuttering, helping him accept that fact that he stutters so he will be less concerned about being identified as a "stutterer"

- working with the people in the child's environment so they will have a better understanding of what the child is experiencing. We will address these strategies more fully in Chapter 7.

You may also need to consider a variety of creative scheduling options until the child's concerns about being identified by his peers have diminished. For example, it may be possible to see the child before classes begin, after classes end, during study time, or during homeroom time. Concerns about being called out of class can also be minimized if the child is able to leave class and come to therapy on his own rather than being called out of the class via the intercom or by the speech therapist waiting at the door of the classroom. This option also has the added benefit of encouraging independence in therapy and helping the child take greater responsibility for his own treatment.

No matter what you do to address this situation, it is imperative that you work to address the issues underlying the child's reluctance to let people know he attends speech therapy. Over time, you can help to decrease the child's feelings of embarrassment and shame that may keep him from being open about his speech. The goal is to empower children to accept stuttering, and, ultimately, to be proud of the fact that they are taking control of their speech by learning new skills in therapy. Of course, this does not happen overnight. Still, you must not enable children to hide their stuttering or the fact that they go to speech therapy, for this will only contribute to their long-term concerns about their speech.

What If Stuttering Isn't the Only Issue?

Numerous research studies have shown that children who stutter are more likely than children who do not stutter to exhibit concomitant speech and language disorders (e.g., Bloodstein 1995, St. Louis & Hinzman 1988). Most common among these concomitant problems is speech sound or articulation disorders, which may co-occur with stuttering for as many as 30% to 40% of children who stutter (Wolk et al. 1993; Yaruss, LaSalle, et al. 1998). Language disorders, oral-motor disorders, cognitive disorders, and other fluency disorders such as cluttering may also occur with a higher prevalence than in the population of typically fluent children.

School-age children who stutter may be less likely to experience concomitant disorders than preschoolers because of improvements in children's speech and language that occur as they continue to develop. Regardless of a child's age, however, the presence of a concomitant disorder can impact treatment considerably. Children who exhibit both stuttering and a speech sound or language disorder may require a longer duration of treatment (Conture et al. 1993). They may also be more likely to experience negative reactions from listeners who may have difficulty understanding their speech, in addition to questions about their fluency. Therefore, you must be prepared to actively address concomitant disorders in children who stutter.

When do I address articulation and/or language disorders?

Perhaps the most common question we are asked about concomitant articulation disorders is "When do I treat them?" Often, this question carries with it the following implication: "I want to treat the articulation because I know I can make progress there," though many SLPs acknowledge the very real possibility that the stuttering even may "get worse" or more noticeable while they are working on the speech sounds.

Indeed, several researchers have commented on the fact that some preschoolers seem to begin stuttering while they are receiving therapy for articulation or language disorders (Bernstein Ratner 1995, Hall 1977). For school-age children, the impact of articulation therapy on stuttering is less clear; however, it does seem reasonable that you want to be careful about giving the child who stutters the message that he is not good at speaking or that he needs to speak in a specific, precise way, as is often done in "traditional" articulation therapies (Conture 2001). Thus, treating concomitant disorders must be done cautiously, and with appropriate consideration to the child's needs in both areas (Logan & LaSalle 2003).

When working with children who stutter who also have concomitant speech sound disorders, you are faced with three basic options:

1. Treat the stuttering first.
2. Treat the speech sounds first.
3. Treat both disorders simultaneously.

As with all aspects of stuttering, there is no "hard and fast" rule that must be applied in all cases. Still, it is important to recall this fact: *speech sound disorders are relatively stable from day to day, while stuttering is subject to dramatic swings in frequency and severity due to the variability of the disorder.* Because of the possibility that stuttering might become more severe in a relatively short period of time, we prefer to initiate treatment by addressing the stuttering, even if in a preliminary fashion, before initiating treatment for the articulation concerns. In other words, we like to begin the process of helping the child come to terms with stuttering and minimize the likelihood of strong negative reactions to stuttering. Then, in the more open context of a greater understanding of the speaking process and greater willingness to "talk about talking," we can begin to address the articulation concerns. This sequence allows us to help the child come to terms with the fact that he has a communication disorder before requiring him to make a significant commitment to practicing changes in his speech production.

It is worth noting that a school-age child with a lingering articulation disorder may be likely to experience the same negative reactions and concerns about his speaking ability as a child with a persistent stuttering disorder (Bothe 2002). Therefore, aspects of the therapy process that are aimed at improving comfort with communication, acceptance of speech errors, etc., will also be beneficial for school-age children with concomitant articulation disorders.

For children with language disorders, your choice is similar. In this case, you may also want to consider whether the child's language formulation concerns may be contributing to the fluency breakdowns. Ultimately, you will need to address the fluency to ensure that the child's stuttering does not increase during the course of the language treatment and you may find benefits to treating both disorders simultaneously.

What about second languages and cultural diversity?

Increasingly, SLPs are working with children and families from various cultural backgrounds, and we have all learned that the child's cultural background must be considered when planning individualized treatment programs (Battle 1998). It is not clear, however, exactly how multicultural factors affect the treatment of children who stutter.

There is some evidence that the prevalence of the stuttering disorder may be different in various cultural groups, with a higher prevalence among African-American students (Gillespie & Cooper 1973) and lower prevalence among Hispanic-Americans (Leavitt 1974). Also, some have suggested that children who are learning English as a second language, or children who are multilingual, may exhibit different characteristics in their stuttering than monolingual children (Van Borsel et al. 2001). Still, the prevalence of stuttering across cultures is believed to be in the general vicinity of 1%, and the impact of various cultural and linguistic factors on a child's stuttering is highly individualized (Tellis & Tellis 2003).

Of course, multicultural issues play a role in the diagnosis and treatment of all disorder areas SLPs work with. Fortunately, numerous resources are available detailing the specific issues that may be affected by the child's background and culture. Areas to consider include:

- the family's beliefs about the role of the family and the role of the clinician in intervention
- use of terminology for describing disorders
- how the family perceives the gender and age of the child *and* the clinician
- use of formal titles when addressing family members
- difficulties that may be experienced due to language barriers

In addition, some topics that are particularly relevant to children who stutter include:

- the family's perception of stuttering as a communication disorder
- the appropriateness of direct eye contact within the culture
- how individuals and families deal with issues such as embarrassment or shame
- the amount of effort that is expected of children in therapy

It is difficult to provide specific guidelines about what adaptations might need to be made in therapy for a given child, and you need to be cautious about over-generalizing cultural beliefs or stereotypes to all of the children from a particular cultural group. Because treatment plans are targeted at each child's specific needs, you must work with the individual family to determine their attitudes about these issues.

What if the child has "real" emotional issues?

Although we have outlined a number of useful strategies for helping children who stutter overcome negative affective and cognitive reactions to stuttering, we do not believe that you have to "go it alone" when helping children deal with their feelings. Some children may actually have emotional reactions that are too great or too entrenched for you to address effectively. In such cases, we feel it is appropriate and, indeed, necessary, for you to partner with other professionals who have specific training in helping children or families deal with emotional issues. We never hesitate to at least consult with mental health professionals, school psychologists, or social workers if we feel that a child exhibits affective or cognitive reactions to his stuttering that will interfere with his progress in speech therapy.

In order to achieve success in your partnerships with other professionals, you must educate them about stuttering. Key issues that we cover include:

- the variability of stuttering
- the fact that stuttering is not a psychological or emotional problem
- the fact that there is no easy solution or cure for stuttering
- the notion that changing stuttered speech can be difficult for the child

By partnering with other professionals who are knowledgeable about stuttering, you can strive to help all of the children you work with to better cope with their stuttering and achieve greater success in therapy.

When Will This Be Fixed?

Addressing a stuttering disorder takes time. Many adults who stutter report that they have been in speech therapy numerous times throughout their lives and that they view dealing with their speech as an ongoing issue (Yaruss et al. 2002). For children who stutter, the long-term nature of speech therapy may be frustrating. They may wonder when it will be "fixed" and when they won't have to come to therapy anymore. Parents, too, want to know when their child's speech will improve to the point where he can communicate more freely or simply more fluently. It is important for you to be prepared to answer children's and parents' questions about the time course of therapy, for it can help everybody involved in the situation to have more patience. They will be able to accept the nature of stuttering therapy more readily if they have a sense about what to expect and if they know when they will see the progress they are hoping for.

When will he get better?

When parents and teachers ask when a child will get better, they are typically asking when he will be more fluent. In answering this question, you have the opportunity to educate the people in the child's environment about the true nature of the stuttering disorder. This does not mean you should tell them "there's no cure for stuttering" or "he will always stutter." To the family, this may translate to "he'll never get better" which is far from true. Instead, you must be sure that everybody in the child's life understands the many ways in which the child will "get better" that do not necessarily involve the development of completely fluent speech. The child will participate more in activities, he will feel better about himself, he will become more accepting of his speaking difficulties, he will develop into a better communicator, and, of course, his fluency *will* improve and the severity of his stuttering *will* decrease. All of these are signs of improvement that everybody in the child's environment must be certain to recognize and value. If others do not value these gains, it will be difficult for the child to value them.

Because the process of "getting better" has many different facets, the question of *when* he will get better is not always easy to answer. The child will make progress on different aspects of his therapy at different rates and at different times during his overall development. Because you are not always working on all goals at the same time, you should not expect progress in all areas at all times. Thus, in order to answer this question for parents and teachers, you must present the "bigger picture" of dealing with stuttering over a lifetime, while at the same time making sure that you present reasonable expectations. By showing the child and his family that progress occurs in many domains, both in the short term and in the long term, you can be a consistent, calming, knowledgeable presence that helps to bring a sense of order and hope that the child *will* achieve success.

Planting the seeds

If you are going to be able to effectively communicate faith, hope, and optimism about the future to the child and his family, you must feel it yourself. Because changes in speech occur over time, and because a child may work with several different clinicians during their lifetime, you may not be the clinician who ultimately gets to see the child achieve the success you have envisioned

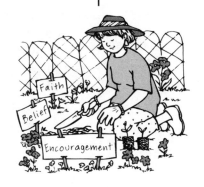

for him. In fact, you may only get to see a brief glimpse of the overall process that he will go through as he learns to successfully manage his speech and his communication attitudes.

For some clinicians, this may be discouraging. For many other disorders we work with, such as articulation disorders, we have the reward of seeing the child's speech improve during the course of therapy. For stuttering, however, the fruit of our labor might not be seen until well after the child has moved on to another clinician. This is when we must cultivate the art of faith. We may never get to see each child run for student council president or give a speech at high school graduation. We must have faith, however, that we are planting the seeds for this possibility for every child we work with. Whatever foundation we can give children while they are in our care will serve them well as they move to other schools, transition in and out of therapy, and even as they grow into young adults.

Taking a "long-term" view

We are not the only one who must take a long-term view of the child's progress in stuttering therapy. Teachers, parents, siblings, administrators, and friends must all recognize that the child's success will unfold over time. Of course, stuttering is not the only aspect of a child's development for which this is true. *All* aspects of a child's development, from athletic skill to reading and writing ability, to knowledge about mathematics, to interpersonal skills, to physical coordination, develop over time. Parents do not expect a child to have a seventh grade reading ability when he is in third grade. Similarly, they should not expect him to have advanced skills for coping with stuttering before he is ready.

It is understandable why parents may feel some urgency about the child's progress in therapy sooner rather than later. Stuttering is not fun to do or to watch. Still, as the child and his family become more comfortable with stuttering, they will gain some tolerance for the disfluencies in the child's speech. They will find it easier to take a long-term view of progress in therapy, and their sense of urgency will diminish.

When you learn to take a long-term view of dealing with stuttering, you can serve as a model for not only the child who stutters, but for all those who may still be waiting for that "fix" of perfect fluency. Fortunately, you have many tools at your disposal to help families adopt this long-term view. You can draw parallels between the child's progress in therapy and his progress in other aspects of development. You can use analogies to describe the process of therapy (e.g., the "journey" analogy described in Chapter 5, pages 203–205). And, perhaps even more importantly, you can help parents and others visualize the child's future success, 5 years, 10 years, or even 20 years in the future. Because you have faith in the child's ability to overcome the *problem* of stuttering, you can visualize him in positive, successful ways. You can see the child communicating freely, saying the things he wants to say, achieving a degree of comfort with his stuttering, developing the ability to advocate for himself with others, and pursuing the life goals he wants to pursue (and you can help the child learn to create these visualizations too).

Keeping this optimal outcome in mind enables you to weather the short seasons of frustration or relapses the child may experience. This will allow you to help the child move toward the positive, long-term view you hold for him. Sometimes, you may be the only one who can maintain this positive frame of mind, so you need to share your faith and belief in the future with the child and everybody in his environment. Doing this helps to strengthen trust and hope for those who do not yet believe it themselves.

Expansion Activities ——————————————

Use this sheet to take responsibility as you become your own speech manager.

Name _____ Goal _____ Bring this back on _____

Where will I do this? _____ Challenge ("Taking a Risk") Activity, if any _____

_____

	Who did I practice with?	What did we do?	How long did I practice?
Sunday			
Monday			
Tuesday			
Wednesday			
Thursday			
Friday			
Saturday			

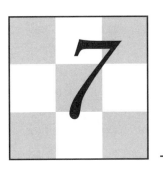

7

No Child Is an Island

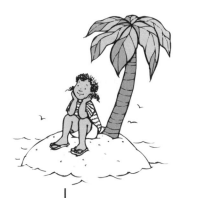

So far in this book we have focused primarily on the needs of children who stutter. We have talked about how to help a child change her observable stuttering behaviors, and we have explored how to help the child minimize her negative affective, behavioral, and cognitive reactions to stuttering so she can communicate as effectively as possible. To achieve optimal success in treatment, we must address more than just the child who stutters; we must also consider other people in the child's world. In this chapter, therefore, we focus on the needs of the people in the child's environment, such as the families, teachers, and peers. We will also discuss the impact these people may have on the child and the child's communication.

How Do I Work with the Parents?

Numerous authors have commented on the importance of working with the entire family when helping children who stutter (Andrews & Andrews 2000, Gottwald & Hall 2002, Zebrowski & Schum 1993). Although it is primarily the child who needs to make changes in speech and communication attitudes, the family also has work to do. Furthermore, the family can play an important role in helping the child achieve and maintain the changes she makes in therapy. They will have difficulty doing this, however, if they are not "on board" with the goals of therapy, and if they do not fully understand the broad-based nature of the stuttering disorder.

Clinicians often lament the fact that it is difficult to have much contact with the parents when working in the school setting. Parents are not available to bring the children to therapy or receive regular updates about the child's progress. Sometimes, it seems that the only times we see parents are during IEP meetings or when there is a problem (e.g., when the parents are concerned that the child has not made enough progress in therapy). If the parent does not wish to participate in the therapy process, there is relatively little we can do other than provide information and encouragement through the child. Still, there are many parents who do want to know what they can do for their children. There is much that we can do to help those parents even without consistent, direct contact.

What do parents need from us?

Before we can meaningfully address the ways parents can help children who stutter, we must first consider the parents' needs. As children make progress in therapy, they experience reductions in the frequency of stuttering, to be sure, but they also learn to accept the fact that they stutter. Parents, on the other hand, do not typically have the benefit of therapy to help them learn that it is "okay to stutter." They may remain "stuck" with the same concerns about their child's speech that they had at the beginning of treatment and they do not make the same progress as their child does.

In a private setting, clinicians may be able to have parents join the child for desensitization exercises. Or they may be able to spend time counseling and educating parents to help them achieve understanding and acceptance of stuttering. In school settings, this is harder to do. The responsibility for educating parents and helping them on their own road to acceptance falls more and more to the child. The younger the child is, the harder this may be to do; however, it is not impossible.

Ultimately, what parents need most is the assurance that their child will be okay. They may assume that the only way for this to happen is for the child to become fluent. In most cases, however, the parents' true goals are not so much about perfect fluency as they are about helping the child communicate freely and effectively without shame or fear. As with all things, parents want their children to be happy, healthy, and well-adjusted.

Our task, then, is to help parents realize that their child *can* achieve these ultimate goals even if some stuttering remains. You cannot convince them of this fact through persuasion or cajoling. You must help them come to this understanding gradually and over time, *just as you do with the child.* And, just like the child, parents will never achieve this goal if they do not develop some acceptance of stuttering.

Thus, our goals for working with the parents become quite similar to our goals for working with the child. The parents should be aware that their child can learn to manage her stuttering so it does not have a negative impact on her ability to achieve her goals in life. They need to learn that it *is* possible for their child to speak freely even if she does stutter. And they need to learn that their child *can* get to the point where stuttering does not cause embarrassment, shame, or fear.

How do I get the parents "in tune"?

Changes in attitudes do not come automatically for the child in therapy, and they do not come automatically for parents either. If parents have difficulty understanding the importance of desensitization exercises, practicing stuttering, and accepting some disfluency as part of the overall definition of success, this can undermine the child's attempts to work toward acceptance. It can also lead to tension between the child and the parents, as well as between the parents and you.

One way we can help parents focus on the goals of therapy is to ask them the following question: "Assuming that your child *does* continue stuttering, what would you like her life to be like in five years?" Nearly every time, the answer will have more to do with overall satisfaction in life rather than specific fluency in speech. When we show them how our therapy procedures are actually focused on these broader goals, many of their concerns are eased.

Parents also need to see ample evidence of the fact that the child *is* able to communicate more freely and more effectively than before treatment. The child can be our best ally as we seek to help parents come to terms with stuttering *if* she keeps her parents informed of the progress she is making. Children in therapy should explain the following concepts to their parents:

- what stuttering is
- what happens with their speech when they stutter
- what their speech management strategies are
- how well the strategies work in different situations
- which speaking situations are easier and which are harder, and why
- what things they do and do not do because of their stuttering
- how they feel when they stutter and when other people react negatively to their stuttering
- what changes they are experiencing in their speech, their attitudes, and in their abilities to communicate

If the parents are kept informed, they will be better able to recognize their child's progress. This will help them get "in tune" with the goals for helping the child improve her communication.

Parents ask: Why is my child still stuttering?

By now, you will recognize that school-age children who stutter are likely to continue stuttering to some extent even when therapy is successful. If parents understand the goals of therapy, then they too will recognize this, and they will be able to help the child achieve a balanced outcome from therapy. If they do not understand this, however, they will want to know why the child has been in therapy for so long without "getting rid of" the stuttering.

Education about the broad-based nature of the stuttering disorder and discussion of the hard truth that there is no cure for stuttering is essential for helping parents come to terms with their child's speech difficulties. Although parents may find this uncomfortable, disappointing, and frustrating, they will never be able to move on to acceptance without first hearing the truth. We must approach this topic delicately, of course, but we must not let fear prevent us from providing an honest assessment of the child's prognosis. It is important for parents to realize that their child's speech *can* improve in therapy, and that the child can learn to manage her stuttering successfully.

A key aspect of helping parents make this transition is making sure they understand that the child will not necessarily continue stuttering *in the same way* throughout her life. This is particularly true if a child is going through a stage where she is having greater difficulty, as is commonly the case when parents contact clinicians to ask about the child's progress in therapy. They may see an increase in severity as a permanent problem rather than a reflection of the variable nature of stuttering. Also, they may tend to assume the worst about the child's reactions to stuttering instead of remembering that it is possible for the child to learn to deal with the fact that she stutters.

Parents need to be informed about the child's progress in therapy. As we described previously, the child is the best person to provide this information. We also need to be sure that we highlight specific aspects of the child's success that extend beyond the production of fluent speech. As part of this goal, we must help parents recognize that children cannot be expected to use their speaking strategies all the time. Children are most successful at applying speaking strategies when they use them on an "as needed" basis. If parents do not understand this, they may expect the child to use her speaking strategies more frequently than she can, or more frequently than she wants to. Ultimately, this may cause the child and family to become discouraged about her progress.

Why are the parents nagging her?

Not surprisingly, many parents of children who stutter just want their children to be able to speak more fluently. Parents may be thrilled when their child learns speaking strategies such as easy starts that help her increase fluency. They see that when the child uses the techniques, she is more fluent. To the parents, then, it makes sense for her to use the techniques as often as possible. They also recognize that she often forgets to use the strategies. As a result, they want to remind her to modify her speech. They see that when they remind her to use her strategies and she starts using them again, her speech fluency increases further. An apparent side benefit of such reminders is that it helps the parents feel like they are doing something useful and proactive to help their child with her speech.

Given the seemingly positive benefits of such reminders, it is easy to see why some parents become overzealous in their attempts to help the child use her speaking strategies. In many cases, it also doesn't take long for the child to grow tired of frequent reminders. Rather than feeling like her parents are helping, the child may feel like her parents are nagging. Tension within the family can be the unfortunate result. (This is especially true if parents correct the child in public. This often happens because parents want their child to "show off" her fluency skills in public situations. Public reminders may also be more likely if the parents are feeling embarrassed or ashamed about the child's stuttering.)

To reduce the risk that the parents will turn into the "stuttering police" (Murphy 1989), we need to make sure the parents know just how hard it is for the child to use speaking strategies. First, parents should be taught how to use the techniques through various collaborative strategies such as handouts sent home with the child and homework exercises in which the child teaches the parents about the techniques. Then parents should be encouraged to practice the techniques right along with the child. This not only helps the child engage in more frequent practice; it also helps to temper parents' enthusiasm as they learn how difficult the techniques are to apply.

Ultimately, some parents who are being too strict in their requirements for speech modifications may need to be told that they should not remind the child to use strategies. Of course, any such restrictions on the parents' behavior should be negotiated between the parents and child. You can help the family find a solution by facilitating this process and making sure that both the parents and the child have a responsibility in the agreement.

A key principle in working with parents of preschool children can be applied to help with overzealous parents of school-age children. Rather than telling their child what they want her to do, parents should instead be required to *show* the child what they want. Thus, if the parents want the child to use more easy starts, then they must use them themselves. If they want the child to reduce tension, then they must demonstrate pseudo-stuttering and modify their pretend tension. By requiring the parents to use the techniques in the real world right along with the child, we can help the parents understand that it is difficult to remember to use modifications all the time. And, any added practice they encourage the child to do in this way is not as likely to be perceived as nagging. In the end, the parents learn more about stuttering and the child gains the opportunity to improve her speech management skills.

What are the parents telling her at home?

As the child begins to experience greater success in therapy, the parents will be eager to offer praise for her accomplishments. Of course, we believe it is good for parents to praise their children. At the same time, we believe that parents need to carefully consider the messages they are sending to the child when they do (or do not) offer praise related to the child's speech.

Because of the affective and cognitive reactions the child may have to her stuttering, comments that are intended to offer praise and support for a job well done can easily be misunderstood. For example, when a child speaks fluently while reading aloud or giving a presentation in class, the parent or teacher may say "you did so great at that!" On the surface this statement seems harmless, for, indeed, the child did do well. If the child has concerns related to self-confidence or self-esteem, however, she may also wonder what the parent would have said if she had stuttered during the presentation. If fluent speech is great, then what is stuttered speech?

The tendency to praise a child more for her fluent speech than her stuttered speech may also be due to the fact that stuttering behaviors are highly variable. There are many times that the child speaks fluently even though she actually did not expect to, or when she did not use any techniques to achieve that fluency. We have two primary concerns with this situation. First, if a parent, clinician, or teacher praises a child's speech only when she is fluent, they run the risk of sending the child the message that fluent speech is the only form of speech that is acceptable. Second, if the people offer praise for fluency in these situations, then the child may not actually know what she did to earn that praise. If she did not specifically try to manage her speech in that situation, then her fluency was, essentially, accidental. This is not a bad thing; however, she cannot try to duplicate her performance to increase her fluency in another situation because she does not know what she did to be more fluent. Again, the praise of fluency sends a mixed message to the child. This can increase her sense of anxiety, shame, or guilt because she does not know what she did to gain that fluency.

As a result, we prefer to teach people to praise the child's *effort*, not the child's *outcome*. In other words, parents can praise the child for attempting to use her speaking strategies (something she has more control over) rather than praising the child for fluency (something she may have less control over). Of course, if the child uses strategies and they help her increase her fluency (as they typically should), then they can praise both the effort and the outcome, pointing out that the child is becoming quite good at using the strategies. This helps to specifically reinforce the lesson we want the child to learn. In essence, the parents can send a more helpful message: When you choose to modify your speech, you can. This will help you speak more easily and, in many cases, more fluently.

Another important way to help parents avoid sending mixed messages is to ensure that they praise the child for progress in *all* aspects of her management of stuttering. In addition to praising the child for using the strategies, she should also be praised for her ability to:

- accept stuttering
- speak freely and to say what she wants to say (rather than avoiding speaking because of the fear of stuttering)
- enter difficult speaking situations
- manage physical tension during fluent and stuttered speech
- communicate successfully regardless of the amount of stuttering in her speech

In this way, parents can play a helpful role in reinforcing all of the strategies that the child is learning in therapy rather than focusing too narrowly on the child's fluency and sending the message that they do not accept the child's speech.

Myth: *"If she only tries hard enough, she can beat this thing."*

Parents who do not understand the goals of treatment for school-age children who stutter may continue to push the child to work on her speech, even if she has reached a point where further changes (at that time) are unlikely. They may be unwilling to accept a plateau in the child's performance, or they may not recognize when the child has achieved as much change in her speech as she is able to at that time. As a result, they may continue to press her to practice and use speaking strategies with the hopes that her fluency will reach "normal" levels. This nagging, frustration, and added pressure may actually reduce the child's overall performance.

While it is certainly true that the child who practices speech and attitude modifications diligently will achieve greater success than the child who does not practice, the belief that the child can overcome stuttering if she simply tries hard enough does not reflect what we know about stuttering or about human behavior and ability in general. In addition to educating parents about stuttering, we may also need to tell parents that attaining success is not simply a matter of trying harder or practicing more. As with all skills, children will reach a level where they have put in all of the effort they are willing to put in for the benefit they receive. Additional pressure to practice or reminders to use strategies will not result in added fluency, for the child will have reached a level that is acceptable to her—even if that acceptable level does not mean perceptibly normal speech.

There are many analogies we can use to get this point across to parents. One example is sports ability. Although everyone can improve their abilities to play golf with added practice and effort, there comes a point at which players may not choose to continue striving because they are satisfied with the levels of proficiency they have achieved. They may practice enough to maintain their current levels of ability, but they may be unlikely to push harder to achieve the "next" levels because of the effort that would be required.

Another pertinent analogy is academic skills. In the acquisition of math skills, students can improve their knowledge of math through practice, effort, and study; however, few people would suggest that all children be required to put in enough practice, effort, and study to be able to become proficient at advanced calculus.

Parents may need to recognize that the child's natural abilities play an important role in determining the child's progress. As with the golf analogy, it may be possible for a "weekend golfer" to compete on a professional level—if he practiced 24 hours a day, seven

continued

days a week. In contrast, a true professional golfer might need only a few hours of practice each day to maintain and refine his skills. In this case, the difference in natural ability results in a dramatic difference in the time investment that is required to reach the highest level of performance. This level of commitment quickly becomes unrealistic for the weekend golfer, just as constant practice and performance is unrealistic for the child who stutters.

The bottom line is that parents need to realize (a) the difficulties involved in changing speech, (b) the child's concerns about her speech will diminish as she progresses through the desensitization components of therapy, and (c) that as "perfect" or "normal" fluency becomes less important to the child, successful communication becomes more possible.

Whose problem is it anyway? Whose *speech* is it anyway?

There is much parents can do to support their child in dealing with stuttering. Ultimately, however, it is the child who needs to come to terms with the disorder. This realization may be difficult for parents to accept, for they generally want to help their child as much as possible. Parents need assurance that they are doing "all they can" to ensure that their child has the best possible opportunity to overcome the difficulties associated with stuttering.

Until parents come to the realization that the disorder actually belongs to the child and not to themselves, it will be difficult for them to let go and allow their child to deal with stuttering in her own way. Because there is no cure for stuttering, the child will have to learn to deal with her stuttering throughout her lifetime. The skills she learns as a child will provide the foundation for later success as an adult. Because stuttering is so individualized, different people need to find the solutions that work for them. Thus, each child needs to have the opportunity to experiment with different strategies for dealing with stuttering in order to find what helps her achieve her greatest success in communication. Again, this means that the parents may need to give her space to find that success. And they will need to respect the choices she makes in reacting to her speaking difficulties. This is particularly true as the child grows older.

Sometimes the child's way of dealing with stuttering is to work hard in therapy and thoroughly learn speaking strategies so she can speak as fluently as possible when she wants to. Other times, however, the child's way of dealing with stuttering may be to use management techniques sparingly and focus on acceptance and speaking freely in most situations. Not surprisingly, parents may find it easier to accept the first example than the second example; however, both are equally valid options. The older the child grows, the more important it is for the parents to respect the child's choices, whatever they may be.

A child can prepare her parents to recognize that she is taking ownership of her speaking difficulties in several ways. She can thoroughly educate her parents about stuttering and stuttering management techniques. She can remind them of the amount of effort involved in managing speech. And she can specifically demonstrate that she can speak freely and communicate effectively without worrying about her stuttering. As the parents see the child's success, they will be less likely to be concerned about whether she is making the right choices in managing her communication disorder.

The child's fine; her family needs treatment!

Throughout this chapter, we have discussed ways of helping parents who are having trouble accepting their child's stuttering. Of course, this is not always the case; many times, parents are supportive of their child's efforts to both manage fluency and accept stuttering. In such cases, the family can play a very helpful role facilitating the child's development of successful communication. Nevertheless, there are many parents who need help to achieve this level of acceptance and support.

In working with parents, it is important to remember that the child has had the benefit of speech therapy to help her achieve acceptance of her stuttering. The parents, unfortunately, have not, unless you and the child make specific efforts to ensure that the parents have the opportunity to grow in their understanding and acceptance of the child's speaking difficulties. Without such efforts, you may find that the child is fine, but the family still wants her to be in therapy.

This is a particularly difficult situation, for you are often obligated to accommodate the parents' wishes and keep the child in therapy. Still, if the child has already achieved the goal of effective communication, she may not have any meaningful goals to address other than to continue practicing. In such cases, perhaps the best that can be done is for the therapy to focus on helping the child learn to advocate for herself and educate those in her environment (including the parents) about stuttering and about the progress she has already made in therapy.

Some may say that it is harmless to keep a child in therapy that she does not really need, pointing out that she may actually make further progress in refining her speech modification skills. This is certainly true, and if the child does not mind being in therapy, there is no problem with writing goals that focus on the child's remaining areas of need. (In fact, this is no different from any other stage of therapy.) The problem only arises when the child does not wish to be in therapy, either because her stuttering is no longer an issue of concern for her, or because she has reached a plateau which, for the time being, prevents her from investing additional effort in learning speech modifications or accepting stuttering. When the child's motivation is low, regardless of the reason, she will be very unlikely to make notable progress in therapy. This may contribute to the parents' concerns about the child's speech, and it may cause the child to become frustrated with having to go to therapy, thereby reducing her progress even further. In such cases, it may be worth talking to the child and family about taking a temporary break from therapy so the child can re-evaluate her goals for treatment and apply her greatest effort at those times when she is most likely to make progress. Again, however, this solution will require the parents to be on board for the goals of therapy. They will also need to be able to recognize the child's progress across a wide variety of relevant domains.

How Do I Work with Teachers?

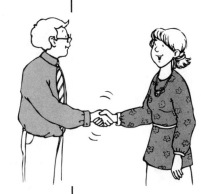

Traditionally, teachers have been "left out of the loop" when it comes to being thoroughly educated about the nature of stuttering or being effectively integrated into a student's therapy. This may particularly be true when a child is being treated in the private sector. No matter what setting you work in, however, it is important to find ways to both educate and collaborate with the teachers of children who stutter.

In the initial stages of developing collaboration with a child's teacher, it may seem to you as if you are "doing all the work." The majority of the information, suggestions, and guidance are provided to the teacher, and it may seem like the teacher has relatively little to contribute to the collaborative process. Over time, however, it will become clear that whatever you give will pay off in the future, and that any such collaboration works to the benefit of the child. A teacher who understands the facts about stuttering and the nature of stuttering treatment can be a strong ally for a child who stutters. The teacher can have a significant positive impact on the child's communicative, social, and academic success, both inside and outside of the classroom. When you put forth the effort to help create this atmosphere, the child's stuttering treatment goals are more easily transferred to situations outside of the therapy room.

Educating teachers about stuttering can also yield significant benefits for you. Having a trained set of eyes (or ears) that can help you learn about the child's experiences in the classroom makes your job easier. This can be particularly useful if you do not have access to the classroom due your clinical setting or because of time constraints. When you collaborate with teachers, they can monitor the child's communication in the school setting and report key information that will help to make therapy more effective. For example, educated teachers can observe the types of disfluencies a child exhibits in the classroom. They can also monitor and report whether a child is transferring techniques learned in therapy. Finally, educated teachers can provide first-hand information about whether a child is exhibiting avoidance behaviors in a salient real-world setting. To help you develop relationships with teachers and educate them about stuttering, you can use a teacher training module such as the one in Appendix 7C, pages 277–287.

Because teachers are such an important part of a child's communicative environment, you must find ways to include them in a child's therapy (Gottwald & Hall 2002, Zebrowski & Cilek 1997). In the next section, we will outline some specific strategies that have helped us effectively integrate teachers into our treatment plan. Of course, there are many more ways to work with educators to help children who stutter. We have simply provided some beginning steps that can then be supplemented or adapted for any therapeutic setting.

Teachers want to help, but they don't know what to do.

It is safe to say that most teachers are in the profession of education because they want to help children. When a teacher has a child who stutters in her classroom, she probably wants to help. In all likelihood, however, she does not have the information or tools she needs to make a positive difference. And, in many cases, the teacher may hold misconceptions about children who stutter (Lass et al. 1992).

A teacher who is educated about stuttering can be a very helpful liaison between the therapy room and the classroom. There are three primary areas where we want teachers to develop their knowledge about stuttering.

1. We want teachers to understand the nature of stuttering, including the specific behaviors exhibited by children who stutter and, in particular, the fact that stuttering varies from day to day and from situation to situation.

2. Teachers need to understand what is involved in stuttering therapy, including the fact that the goals of therapy do not necessarily include "perfectly" fluent speech.

3. Teachers must be able to appreciate the importance of the covert aspects of stuttering, including the child's feelings and beliefs about stuttering, as well as the signs that indicate that a child may be using avoidance strategies.

If teachers can understand these three facts, it will help to reduce confusion that arises when teachers hear the child being fluent one day but not the next, when they report that children "don't stutter much in the classroom" without considering how much the child actually talks, or when they wonder why the child "hasn't made any progress" in learning to speak more fluently.

You can help teachers and other educators acquire this knowledge by highlighting the fact that *stuttering is more than just stuttering*. Teachers may focus primarily on the speech behaviors they can easily see, and they may overlook some of the less visible, but equally important, factors that contribute to the child's experience of stuttering. You can also highlight the fact that *stuttering therapy is more than just therapy for stuttering*. A teacher who understands the broad-based nature of stuttering therapy will have more realistic expectations for the child. She will also be more likely to recognize the child's efforts at improving communication as a whole rather than focusing only on the number of times the child stutters. Ultimately, this will result in increased opportunities for transfer and maintenance of enhanced communication skills within the classroom setting.

Teachers don't have enough time to let the child talk in class.

If a child stutters frequently or with greater severity, she may need extra time to answer questions or participate in discussions in class. This can be a problem for some teachers, for time pressure is one of the most commonly cited concerns among classroom teachers. You can help this situation by validating the teachers' concerns about the time schedule and by brainstorming with them to identify different ways a child can gain the time she needs to actively participate in her academic environment.

Children who stutter have much to contribute during everyday interactions in the classroom. Unfortunately, many classrooms today are fast-paced and over-scheduled. This atmosphere may increase time pressure on the teacher, as well as on all of the children in the class. It is important for you to talk with teachers about the ways they can increase a child's opportunities for successful communication. It is also important for the child to experience positive feelings about answering questions and making comments during classroom discussions.

Some modifications to the classroom routine can be helpful for both the child and the teacher. For example, a child who stutters can be called upon to answer questions at the beginning of class periods when time pressure is not as great. A teacher can also decrease time pressure by talking with the child and letting her know that she has the time she needs to participate in classroom discussions. Several other suggestions follow that can be implemented in everyday classroom interactions to help the teacher develop a better understanding of the child's needs in the classroom while simultaneously helping the child to communicate more effectively.

Answering Questions or Reading Aloud

Teachers may be uncertain about how to help children who stutter during many common classroom tasks, such as answering questions or reading aloud. In fact, teachers often ask us if they should ever call on a child who stutters to answer a question or read aloud in class. In responding, we like to point out that involving the child in regular classroom activities not only provides the child with the opportunity to achieve her educational objectives, it also provides teachers with the opportunity to demonstrate and model (for the child's peers) patient listening and other appropriate reactions to stuttering. We then begin a dialogue with the child's support team (including the child herself) to identify the best ways the teacher and child can handle classroom speaking situations.

Sometimes, teachers wonder if they should call on a child who stutters at all for fear of subjecting the child to greater embarrassment or shame. Oddly, it seems that teachers rarely *ask the child* how she would like the situation to be handled. As with most of the aspects of stuttering, thoughts and feelings about reading aloud or speaking in class are different for different children. Some children—even those who stutter more severely in conversational speech—can read with relative comfort. The reverse is also true, as some children who speak more fluently in conversation may have increased difficulty when reading. You can help the child and teacher identify good strategies by determining the child's level of comfort during reading and learning the teacher's expectations in each subject area. At the same time, you can facilitate the dialogue between the child and teacher to identify strategies that allow both parties to achieve success.

We are often surprised by the creativity our young clients show when we brainstorm with them to identify solutions to the challenges they face. The following suggestions, which come directly from children we have worked with, provide just a few helpful ideas:

- Random Calling: Increased tension can be created when a child who stutters must sit and wait for her turn to talk. One way of decreasing this anticipation pressure is to select children at random rather than simply going in order down the row of chairs. This idea, coupled with the flexibility of "making a plan" that suits the child's needs (perhaps wanting to be called upon first or second) can decrease the anticipation anxiety that a child may be experiencing in the classroom.

Vignette: Answering Questions

Mrs. Jacobs teaches fourth grade. Matt is one of her best students. Matt has been in speech therapy for stuttering since first grade, and he has a great working knowledge of his speech management tools. Matt reports that for the most part, he is "okay" with his stuttering and that he "doesn't let it bother him much."

Mrs. Jacobs has recently reported to the speech therapist, Mr. Rice, that Matt has been repeatedly answering "I don't know" to most of the questions she asks him during classroom discussions. She is concerned about this, as classroom participation affects grading and she believes that Matt really does know the answers.

During subsequent therapy sessions, Mr. Rice discusses classroom participation as a speaking situation on Matt's hierarchy. (See page 202 for a description of hierarchies.) Matt discloses that he is really feeling embarrassed about his stuttering in the classroom and that he is feeling reluctant to talk "in front of the other kids."

Matt and Mr. Rice each complete a problem-solving plan. (See Appendix 7A, page 274 for an example of a problem-solving plan.) They also invite Mrs. Jacobs to fill one out, and they meet together during one of Matt's therapy sessions. Matt explains that he feels rushed to answer questions in class. He reports that the time pressure affects his stuttering and that this is part of what made him start avoiding talking in class.

Together, Mrs. Jacobs and Matt decide that she will give him the extra time he needs by not moving on to another student so quickly. Also, Mr. Rice and Matt resolve to concurrently work on the embarrassment that Matt was experiencing regarding stuttering in front of his classmates.

- Tag-Team Discussions: Communicative pressures can be reduced when the responsibility for a discussion is shared by more than one student. In "tag-team" discussions, a teacher may inform a few students that each is responsible for one part of a selection in reading aloud, or for one part of an answer to a question. This allows the child who stutters to know that she will not be alone in the communication, and this may, in turn, decrease speaking anxiety.

- "Popcorn" Choices: In this discussion method, the teacher chooses the first child to read or answer a question, and then that child chooses the next person. Of course, the teacher must know her class well and be certain of their sense of fairness and camaraderie. For some classrooms, this can be an effective and fun way to include all children in classroom discussions.

There are many ways that you, teachers, and children can work together to address issues in the classroom. It is the SLP's role to support children who stutter in finding their own solutions to the communication problems they face. Thus, you and the child's teachers should be sure to discuss these and other suggestions with the child before implementing them in the classroom.

Oral presentations

Oral presentations can spark anxiety for many children, not just those who stutter. Still, sometimes teachers will want to exempt children who stutter from class presentations, perhaps in an attempt to spare them the anxiety. Our feeling is that children who stutter should always have the same opportunities as other children to participate in class assignments. This means that they should not be automatically exempted from any activity simply due to the fact that they stutter. Thus, those children who can, and who wish to, should be able to give class presentations like their peers.

At the same time, however, teachers must also allow some degree of flexibility to allow children who are not yet able to give whole class presentations so they can complete required tasks in alternate ways. In such cases, you, the teacher, and the child can brainstorm various alternatives that may give the child the opportunity to participate in class without needing to experience significant discomfort associated with the oral presentation. Again, we have been impressed by the creativity of our young clients. Some of their solutions are listed on the next page.

- Have the child give her presentation in a small group setting.

- Have the child give her presentation first (or second) to minimize the buildup of fear and apprehension.

- Allow the child to give her presentation in partnership with another child.

- Remove or extend time limits for the presentation to minimize time pressures.

- Give the child the opportunity to practice her presentation in front of you or the teacher before she faces the class.

- In the most severe cases only, have the child complete an entirely different type of assignment.

It is also important for the teacher and child to consider whether the presentation will be graded on style or content, so the child will know what to expect.

Of course, regardless of the specific solution that is developed in the classroom, your goal should be to help the child get to the point where she can give presentations in class. As with many of the goals in therapy, this is approached through a hierarchy, beginning with easier tasks that the child can complete successfully and gradually moving toward those tasks where the child experiences greater difficulty. An example of a hierarchy prepared by one of our students is shown in the vignette on the next page.

It is worth remembering that although we have suggested that some children who stutter may need adaptations for their oral presentations, this is not always the case. Many children who stutter may not need or want special consideration; they may simply want to be treated the same as everybody else. Therefore, clinicians and the child's teachers must not simply assume that a child needs to do things differently or at a "lower" level simply because she stutters. Instead, like we do for all children, we should set our goals high and then provide the support she may need to achieve those goals.

Recess, Lunch, and the Bus

The classroom is certainly a salient communication situation for school-age children; however, you should not underestimate the importance of the other communication situations a child finds herself in during the day. The playground, the cafeteria, the bus, assemblies, and other social venues are also important for a child who stutters, and a child's success in these situations can play a big role in determining the child's attitudes about herself and her communication.

Some children actually feel less pressure in social situations. These are children who make friends easily and feel that their friends accept their stuttering. As a result, they feel less pressure to "perform" and they are less likely to struggle in their attempts to maintain fluency. For other children, however, social situations cause them to feel greater pressure. These children are less comfortable stuttering openly among their friends or peers, and may be more likely to tense up their speech muscles in their attempts to prevent stuttering. Ultimately, this can lead to greater difficulty with communication, teasing, and many of the other unpleasant consequences of stuttering for school-age children.

Vignette: Classroom Presentations

Mrs. Brown, a sixth grade teacher, approached the speech therapist, Mrs. King, to discuss the upcoming series of oral presentations that will be taking place in her classroom. Mrs. Brown is concerned about her student, Sarah. Sarah exhibits a considerable amount of stuttering during classroom discussions and Mrs. Brown feels that it would be best for Sarah to "opt-out" of the oral presentations, so "she won't be embarrassed in front of her peers."

Sarah knows she has many oral presentations coming up this year, and she has been working on her first one. Sarah and Mrs. King have been working on hierarchies that will help desensitize Sarah to talking in front of the class. Sarah is feeling nervous, but she has a plan in place to make the experiences less threatening.

Sarah's Classroom Speech Plan

Remember: Some steps can take longer than others. Let's take our time to gain confidence and decrease fear at each level.

- Write out comments
- Practice by myself
- Practice out loud (at home)
- Practice with my parents
- Practice alone in classroom
- Practice with a friend in classroom → Before or after class
- Plan with teacher to go first or second
- Do my best!

Mrs. King shares Sarah's hierarchies with Mrs. Brown and discusses with her the goal of having Sarah participate normally in the classroom curriculum. Through these discussions, Mrs. Brown reveals that she finds it hard to watch Sarah struggle when talking in the classroom. Mrs. King validates that this feeling is normal and reassures Mrs. Brown that the goal of therapy is to decrease the impact stuttering has on Sarah's life. They both agree that Sarah's willingness to participate fully in class assignments is the *true* measure of success in this situation, and that whether she stutters during her presentations or not, she is successful for having faced her fears of speaking to the class.

It is worth noting that classroom teachers are usually not present during these less structured parts of a child's day. Often, volunteers or part-time supervisors, cooks, and bus drivers see a very different side of the child's experiences than teachers see in the classroom. If you wish to help the child in all aspects of her daily life, then you must also educate and collaborate with the school support staff and others who interact with the child. To achieve these goals, you must provide basic education about stuttering, information about how to communicate with children who stutter, and suggestions about how to manage problems that may occur. You must also maintain an open line of communication between the support staff and the classroom teacher if any problems should arise.

Teachers are our allies

Overall, your primary goal in working with teachers should be to develop allies who can not only provide first-hand information about the child's experiences in the classroom, but who can also work with you to brainstorm, select, and implement solutions to the challenging situations the child may face. By partnering with teachers in this way, you can ease many of the child's communication concerns in one of her most important speaking environments, and you can simultaneously reduce any anxiety the teacher may be feeling about how she can help children who stutter in the classroom. The efforts you make to educate teachers will help you and your students well into the future, and the partnerships you develop through advocacy for children who stutter will have benefits for children who exhibit other communication disorders as well.

What About Peers?

As a child approaches the school-age years, she experiences a shift in the nature of her conversational interactions. Prior to entering school, her primary conversational partners are parents and siblings—people who (ideally) understand stuttering and are supportive of the child's development. Once she goes to school, however, the child's primary audience becomes her peers. The older she gets, the more important her peer group becomes. Peers serve not only as conversational partners; they are also role models, judges, and comrades in nearly all of the child's experiences from that point forward in her life. For this

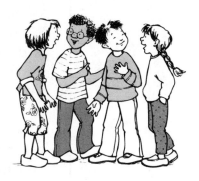

reason, you must consider the potential impact of the child's peer group on her stuttering.

It is important to recognize at the outset that dealing with peers can be a difficult topic for some school-age children. Sometimes, children's difficulties in interacting with peers have little or nothing to do with stuttering. In such cases, we need to seek input from professionals with specific experience in helping children deal with interpersonal relationships. For issues that *are* related to stuttering, however, you can help children who stutter address many of the issues they may face in relating to their peers. Our goal in this section is to review strategies for addressing some of most common concerns expressed by clinicians and children who stutter:

- how to deal with teasing and bullying

- how to appropriately and meaningfully educate the child's peers about stuttering

- how to help the child learn to become an effective, appropriate advocate for herself

As with all aspects of your treatment approach, your goal is to teach the child skills that will serve her throughout life. Learning to deal appropriately with peers is no exception.

Teasing and bullying

Teasing and bullying may be among the toughest obstacles that children who stutter face when interacting with their peers. Research suggests that children who stutter are more likely to experience teasing and bullying than their typically fluent peers (Langevin 1997, Murphy & Quesal 2002). Unfortunately, they may also be less well-equipped to deal with these experiences because of their difficulty with verbal responses.

When approaching the problem of teasing and bullying, it can be helpful to maintain a distinction between comments that are *not* intended to hurt the child (e.g., good-natured teasing or innocent comments about the child's speech) and those statements that *are* intended to cause embarrassment or pain (e.g., inappropriate teasing or bullying). Teasing in and of itself does not necessarily have to be a problem if it is not intended in a hurtful way, *and if it does not feel hurtful to the child*. Many children who have developed comfort with their stuttering have learned how to tease—and be teased—about their speech in a way that is not hurtful.

Bullying, on the other hand, is an entirely different experience, both for the bully and for the child who is being bullied. Bullying occurs when an individual acts in a way that is designed to be hurtful to another individual. Bullies seek to exploit perceived weaknesses among their victims, and they often increase their efforts when they find that they have "hit the mark." Because of their communication difficulties, children who stutter often experience bullying.

The most important thing children, teachers, and families need to know about bullying is that *it is not acceptable*. Nobody deserves to be bullied, and such behavior should not be tolerated by anybody. Research has shown that children who are bullied are more likely to have difficulty with self-esteem, confidence, social interaction, and other key aspects of development (Callaghan & Joseph 1995, Neary & Joseph 1994). Therefore, we cannot take the approach that some bullying is acceptable because "kids are just like that." Instead, we must adopt an attitude of zero tolerance for bullying behaviors. This attitude must come from the top, beginning with parents and teachers. The adults in a child's life must be actively involved in preventing and resolving conflicts associated with bullying.

Understanding bullies

If we intend to help children deal with the effects of bullying, we must understand *why* some children are bullies and where this behavior comes from. The research literature suggests that children become bullies because of their *lack of tolerance for differences* and their own *low self-esteem* (Freedman 2002). Thus, the source of the problem is the bully himself, not the child who is being bullied. Unfortunately, because of their need to feel strong and in control, bullies tend to target children who seem weaker, or who react emotionally to the teasing. Therefore, children who stutter are often a prime target for bullies. To prepare children who stutter to handle bullying and inappropriate teasing, we need to help them recognize that *they* are not the cause of the problem. When we help a child who stutters understand what is behind teasing, it can help her begin to understand that she is not to blame. This can help to increase self-confidence in the child who stutters and, ultimately, shift the "balance of power" between the bully and the child who is being bullied.

The problem of bullying is a part of life for many children who stutter. Before we can begin to help children deal with bullying, we must first get to know more about their experiences, how they have coped with bullying in the past, and the feelings they have experienced as a result of bullying about their stuttering. As we develop a trusting and supportive rapport with the children we work with, they will feel free to share this type of sensitive information. *About Teasing and Bullying* (Appendix 7B, page 276), was created to help us "check in" with a child about her experiences with bullying. This type of activity can create a springboard for many more discussions on the topic of teasing.

Putting an end to bullying

Ultimately, the reasons that children are bullied matter far less than the manner in which a child handles being bullied. Fortunately, children have many options for dealing effectively with the effects of bullying. There are a growing number of helpful resources available that clinicians and other educators can use to teach children the importance of acceptance, and many school districts have already implemented general character education curriculums that help children learn to respect the differences in each other. The psychology, counseling, and social work literature also provides a wealth of options for responding to teasing and bullying. We have provided a number of resources in the reference list (pages 292–301) and there are many others that can help you, parents, teachers, and children deal more effectively with teasing.

There is also literature designed specifically to help the child who stutters. Organizations such as the National Stuttering Association (NSA) have created resources designed specifically to foster acceptance and tolerance of people who stutter. For example, the NSA has produced a poster that teachers can put in their classrooms (not just classrooms with children who stutter) that highlights a variety of differences children may see in each other (e.g., red hair, green eyes, braces, athletic) and explains that these differences are "no laughing matter." The NSA has also prepared a booklet specifically designed to help children who are being bullied. Such efforts by independent organizations as well as school districts may help to decrease the levels of bullying over time. In the meantime, however, you must continue to be diligent in consistently providing support, education, and consistency for both the child who stutters and for the child who bullies.

When a child is being bullied about her stuttering, you can and must get involved. *How* you get involved depends upon the child's wishes, as well as upon the seriousness of the situation. Your ultimate goal is to provide the child with a variety of coping strategies for dealing with bullying and to empower her to handle the situations to the best of her ability. To achieve this goal, you must be prepared to work not only with the child herself, but also with the people in the child's environment.

Educating others

Helping the child learn how to respond to inappropriate comments will go a long way toward reducing the problems associated with bullying; however, by itself, this is not sufficient. Teaching others about stuttering is an important part of our role as clinicians, and an essential aspect of decreasing bullying about stuttering. You can educate others in a variety of ways, and can choose strategies that are most comfortable for the child with whom you are working. In the following paragraphs, we describe a number of different strategies—from less direct to more direct—that will help children who stutter begin the process of learning to educate others about stuttering.

Less direct strategies include going into classrooms to educate students about "what speech teachers do." A teacher or social worker can help classmates understand some of the challenges that are faced by other children, regardless of the specific nature of their differences or disorders. These indirect strategies can provide only general information about the nature of stuttering. A more powerful way to educate peers is to *directly involve the child who stutters* in educating others. Ultimately, the child who stutters will need to develop the ability to educate other people about stuttering, for this is a situation she will face all of her life. We can plant the seeds for the long-term development of this skill early in the therapy process by helping the child learn to educate her peers at school.

A child can be involved in teaching others about stuttering in a variety of ways and at a variety of levels, and it is important to work with the child to determine the most appropriate way for her to provide this education. For example, she can write a note or letter about stuttering to a teacher or to the students in her classroom. She can use assignments given in class (e.g., written assignments that are read to the group) to educate her peers about stuttering. And, for some, the ultimate education for peers can be a classroom presentation about stuttering (Murphy & Quesal 2002). This presentation can be done with or without you in the classroom, but it is always advisable for you to be involved in planning the presentation and providing support for the child before the presentation is scheduled.

A classroom presentation can be considered the pinnacle of desensitization activities for school-age children who stutter. Many children will, at first, express concern and fear about talking with their class about stuttering; however, others will see this as an opportunity to say the things they've always wanted to say about their speech in a situation where they are in control of the class. We have done many of these types of presentations with our young clients, and we always find it to be an enlightening and empowering experience.

When a child is ready to give a presentation about stuttering, you can help her prepare by first discussing the goals she hopes to achieve. Many times, we find that children simply want others to understand that stuttering is not something they are doing on purpose, that it is not their fault, and that simple suggestions, such as "slow down" or "think about what you are saying" do not help them speak more easily. Other times, they may have more specific messages they want to convey, such as what it feels like to stutter or how their stuttering has affected their school work. Following the goal-setting discussions, work with the child to develop an appropriate outline for the presentation. Then brainstorm activities the child can incorporate into the presentation to help her peers truly understand her experiences (e.g., teaching other children how to pseudo-stutter, use speaking strategies such as "easy starts" or "easing out," role-playing common teasing situations). Finally, help the child prepare for the actual presentation by practicing the talk, posing sample questions, and preparing solutions to different problems that may arise. Ultimately, the child can go to her class, tell her peers the things she wants them to know about her speech, and provide needed education for others about stuttering.

Classroom presentations have become a more common component of speech therapy for school-age children who stutter, even those who are being seen by clinicians who work outside of the school settings. In recent years, a growing body of literature has developed that can help children and their clinicians prepare for their presentations. For example, the NSA has prepared a pamphlet that provides a sample presentation outline (Murphy & Reardon 2001).

A well-planned and carefully prepared presentation is always a positive experience for both the child who stutters and her classmates. We are often amazed at how many of the child's peers have questions about stuttering that they never thought they could ask. So many of the children really want to understand what stuttering is all about and what is happening to their friend when she stutters. Through these types of classroom presentations, the myths surrounding the child and the stuttering can be changed into facts, behaviors that seemed weird become understandable, and the child who stutters becomes less of a target for bullying by the other children in the classroom.

Working with the child

Understandably, a child who is being bullied simply wants to find a way to get the bully to stop bullying her. As described above, there are many things you, teachers, and children can do to reduce the likelihood that others will respond to the child who stutters with intolerance. At the same time, however, you must also help children understand that *they cannot directly change the actions of another person.* What they *can* do is change the way they respond to the bully. The goal is to help children select responses that decrease the likelihood that the bullying will continue.

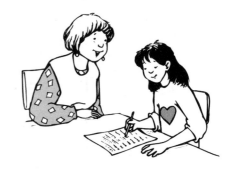

Because bullies tend to pick on children who are weaker physically or emotionally, it is reasonable to conclude that the less emotions a child shows in responding to the bully, the less likely the bully will be to continue his unpleasant behavior. Of course, it will be difficult for the child who stutters to respond to bullying without emotion if she is already feeling embarrassment, fear, or shame about her speech. Therefore, *the foundation for helping a child respond appropriately to bullying and teasing is to help the child become more accepting of her stuttering.* This is accomplished through the exploration and desensitization exercises described in Chapter 4. As the child who stutters becomes less concerned about her stuttering, the bullying and teasing will have less of an effect on her, and it will be easier for her to respond to the bully in a manner that is more likely to reduce the bullying.

In addition to desensitizing the child to stuttering, you can help her deal with bullies by teaching specific strategies for responding when bullying and inappropriate teasing occur. Fortunately, many such strategies are available. Because children's abilities to react to bullying are dependent upon their own self-confidence and self-esteem, however, they must be allowed to individually select the strategies they will use. We cannot "fix" the problem for them or be directly involved in every situation. We can only make suggestions for them to consider and then ask them questions that will lead them toward positive actions and personal empowerment.

As children are exploring different responses to bullying, they must be allowed to say whatever they want and whatever they feel without judgment. Thus, if a child needs to express her desire to respond physically by hitting the bully, she needs to be allowed to say this and consider the implications of such actions so she can be guided toward selecting a more appropriate response (Murphy & Quesal 2002). Similarly, if a child wants to explore the possibility of simply walking away from the bully, she should not be judged as "wimpy" because she is not "standing up for herself." The child will only be able to use a strategy consistently if it feels right to her and if it ultimately helps to reduce the bullying.

It is important to remember that verbal "comebacks" may be very difficult for children who stutter to use effectively. The child may already be fearful or tense in situations where she is being bullied, so it may be even harder for her to maintain fluency. This is another reason we believe it is important for the specific strategies to be selected by the child rather than being determined by you or the parent. *Regardless of which strategies are selected, they should help the child feel good about herself and about how she is handling these situations.* This will help her learn that she can use these strategies in the future to manage the situations she will face throughout her life.

Of course, you can help children explore a variety of alternatives, and you may need to make some initial suggestions to help them think about helpful and effective ways to deal with bullies. Because every child is different, and because children will experience different situations throughout their lives, you should try to provide children with opportunities to brainstorm *many* strategies that they can use. These suggestions may include indirect, nonverbal responses as well as more direct, verbal responses.

Indirect or nonverbal responses are designed to protect the child from the bullying behavior and to remove her from the situation if necessary.

- **Ask for help.** Talk with teachers or playground supervisors so someone can help "watch over" the situation. (If children select this option, it is important to help them recognize that there is a difference between "tattling" and "telling." Tattling is done to get the other person in trouble; telling is asking for help with a situation in an effort to make it better.)

- **Ignore + Self-Talk** Walk away from the bully while reminding yourself of a positive message. For example, "I don't believe what he says. I am okay."

- **Protective Shield** Imagine there is a shield or a bubble surrounding you that makes hurtful words bounce off.

- **Ignore + Imagine + Talk** Walk away from the bully while imagining that you got to tell the bully exactly what you wanted to really say! Know that someday you will be able to do just that. Then talk with someone you trust about what you wanted to say.

Verbal responses are designed to deflect the bully's criticisms in a way that will lead to a reduction of the bullying. They are not designed to hurt the bully in return; they are simply an attempt to let the bully know that the hurtful words did not actually hurt.

- **Agree with the bully** "Yep, I stutter."

- **Ask a question** "Did you think of that by yourself?"

- **Reflect the tease** "Why would you want to say something like that to me?"

- **Use an "I" message** "I don't want you to talk to me like that!"

- **Take it as a compliment** "Thanks for noticing that about me."

- **Walk away WITH PURPOSE** "I don't need this."

- **Say something that is hard to for the bully to respond to** "So?" or "and . . . ?"

- **Compliment the bully** "Yep, I stutter. I wish I could talk like you."

- **Use humor** "Yep, I stutter. That means everything I say is important enough to say twice!"

It is helpful to view these responses to bullying along a hierarchy as you have done with the other aspects of therapy. For example, a child who is fearful about her speech may need to begin with less confrontational and less assertive types of responses to bullying. Then as her ability to effectively handle bullying grows, and as her self-esteem, confidence, and acceptance increases, she will be able to move toward more direct responses.

Finally, it is worth noting that all of the above ideas are ones that are meant to *diffuse* the situation. Often, in their attempts to help children overcome bullying, adults may encourage children to hit back, tease back, or somehow get the bully in trouble. Unfortunately, these types of responses do little to decrease the bullying, and can often lead to an escalation toward inappropriate verbal or physical exchanges. You can help children and their parents work through these situations by being role models for positive responses that diffuse the situation rather than negative reactions that escalate it.

Is She the Only One Who Stutters?

In 2000, the American Speech-Language-hearing Association (ASHA) conducted a survey examining the caseloads of SLPs working in different clinical settings. Results indicated that 80% of school-based therapists reported that they work with children who stutter. Nevertheless, the number of children who stutter on the average clinician's caseloads each year was only 2.4—the lowest of any of 15 disorder areas that ASHA examined.

As a result, even though the true prevalence of stuttering is approximately 1% of the population, many professionals are likely to believe that stuttering is a "low-incidence" disorder compared to other disorders they work with. The perception that stuttering is a low-incidence disorder, combined with the fact that many clinicians have very few children who stutter on their caseloads, contributes to a number of the problems we have addressed in this book (e.g., a general lack of knowledge among many clinicians about stuttering therapy, low confidence in treatment skills).

"She's the only child who stutters in my whole building."

Children who stutter can feel very alone in the school setting. Even though there may be other children who stutter in their school, they may not be the same age and they may not be able to connect with each other in any meaningful way. You can help children who stutter find support in other children who stutter by being a liaison between the children on your caseload. You can create opportunities for children who stutter to interact with one another in at least three ways:

1. Group children together in therapy.

   Even though we believe it is important for children who stutter to receive individual therapy sessions, we also understand that there are caseload considerations that require us to put children who stutter in therapy groups with other children. When grouping is necessary, it is helpful to provide at least some therapy time for children who stutter to be grouped with other children who stutter. It can be a wonderful experience for children who stutter to see how other children who have had similar experiences may have learned to deal with their own stuttering.

Of course, it is not always possible to form homogeneous groups where every child is experiencing the same communication disorder. This is particularly true for stuttering. We have found that groups involving children with different communication disorders can also be beneficial for children who stutter as they can learn helpful coping strategies from other children with speech and language difficulties, even if the specific nature of the disorder is not the same. We say more about grouping children who stutter with children with other communication disorders in Chapter 6 (page 228).

2. Group children together in social events.

   If it is not possible to group children who stutter together in therapy, you can consider bringing them together for occasional fun times that are directed more toward social communication and sharing rather than specific therapy goals and objectives. This can work well for children in the same school, even if the children are different ages or are at different places in their therapies. Of course, this may require more creativity to accomplish if the children come from different schools; however, the benefits of bringing children who stutter together with other children who stutter cannot be underestimated. We have seen older children become role models for younger ones— and, we have also seen young children teach teenagers some new perspectives about how to successfully deal with stuttering!

3. Provide opportunities for children to connect with others outside of school.

   When there are no other children who stutter in a school, or if there are concerns that interactions with other children in the school may not be positive, consider other avenues for encouraging your students to connect with other children who stutter. The best way that we have found for accomplishing this important goal is to partner with support groups for people who stutter, or through carefully chosen and monitored websites. With the help of these outside resources, children can meet others who stutter, either directly or through letters, e-mails, or newsletters. We will say more about support groups in the next section, and a list of helpful resources for linking children who stutter with others is included in Appendix 2A, pages 45–46.

Regardless of the specific strategy that is used, children who stutter must come to understand they are not alone in dealing with their stuttering. Children who stutter learn best from others who have had similar experiences. The feeling of support and camaraderie that they receive from interacting with other people who stutter helps them face many of the issues that may arise as they learn to deal with their stuttering. You can facilitate this process by ensuring that you provide children who stutter with opportunities to share with others and to receive this type of support when they are ready.

They're the only parents on the block with a child who stutters.

Parents, too, may feel like their children are alone in their battles with stuttering. They see that their children are isolated because of their fears about interacting with others, talking on the phone, making friends at school, etc. Furthermore, as the parents look around, they see that other children seem to communicate effortlessly. This can magnify their concerns about their own child's speaking difficulties.

Earlier in this chapter, we outlined several strategies for working with parents of children who stutter. You can do even more to help the families of children who stutter by making sure they understand that their children do not have to face stuttering by themselves. Not only are there other children who stutter in the child's local region; there are also many, many children and adults who stutter throughout the country. You can put children who stutter in touch with other children who stutter so they can see that they are not alone (Bradberry 1997, Reardon & Reeves 2002).

Parents, too, can benefit from meeting other parents of children who stutter. In fact, interaction with other parents often reinforces the messages you have been trying to provide to the parents you work with, and this can help parents feel better about their child's stuttering as well.

"You're not alone" — The value of stuttering support groups

Given that there are substantial benefits to helping children who stutter interact with other children who stutter, it makes sense to incorporate a group component in your treatment as much as possible (Bradberry 1997, Ramig 1993, Reardon & Reeves 2002). To varying degrees, this can be done within the context of therapy as described in this chapter; however, such grouping is not always feasible.

Even if a child can be grouped with other children who stutter in school-based therapy, there is still more that you can do to achieve the important goal of helping children who stutter interact with one another or with other adults who stutter. For example, you might bring your students and families together for a monthly meeting. The focus of the meeting can either be to answer the parents' questions and concerns about their child's therapy or simply to allow parents to provide support to one another.

An easier way of getting people who stutter connected with other people who stutter is to partner with a local stuttering support group in your area. For example, the National Stuttering Association (NSA), which is the largest support group in the United States for people who stutter, has several programs for helping children who stutter and helping their families meet other children who stutter and their families. Events such as youth days, an annual conference, and local youth and teen chapters provide excellent means of helping children who stutter find support from other people who stutter.

As clinicians, we partner with support groups because support groups help us do our jobs better. More importantly, support groups help the children we work with develop the skills they need to carry them on their journeys throughout their lives. The benefits of support cannot be underestimated. The support group environment can reinforce the message that the child is okay and that it is okay to stutter. By meeting with other children who stutter, your students can learn other ways to handle their stuttering. By meeting adults who stutter who have learned to manage their speech effectively, or who have learned to minimize the impact of stuttering on their lives, children can see that they can indeed overcome many of the negative consequences of their stuttering. The support environment provides hope and encouragement, and it helps to prepare children for long-term success by showing them that it is possible for them to maintain the changes they make in therapy and incorporate those changes into their lives.

Helping the Child Advocate for Herself

Given the undeniable influence that parents, teachers, and peers can have on a child's experience of the stuttering disorder, it is imperative that you address the child's environment when working with children who stutter. Nonetheless, in the end, it is the child herself who has to develop the skills she needs to successfully cope with her own stuttering throughout her life. Therefore, in addition to working with the environment, we have to help the child learn to advocate for herself.

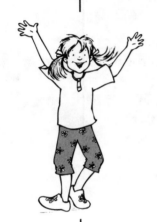

Because there are so many public misconceptions about stuttering, people who stutter need to be able to educate others about stuttering. They need to be able to counter myths and present facts about stuttering in a straightforward way without experiencing embarrassment or shame about the fact that they stutter. To do this, they will need to feel a sense of power over their own lives and over their stuttering. Without this empowerment, children may feel that they are the "victim" of their stuttering. They may feel that there is nothing they or anybody else can do to help them, and this creates barriers that prevent them from effectively dealing with their stuttering.

Becoming empowered

The best way that SLPs and families can counter this sense of victimization about stuttering is to help the child realize that she *can* improve her speech, that she *can* face her fears about speaking, that she *can* communicate effectively, and that she *can* positively affect the environment in which she lives. Note that all of these aspects of becoming empowered to manage stuttering are part of the overall process of therapy we have described throughout this book.

1. **Understanding speaking and stuttering**
   Even during the early school-age years, children can learn about the process of speaking so they will better understand what they are doing when they stutter. We cannot change what we do not understand, so this knowledge is a necessary first step for helping children learn to manage their stuttering over the long term.

2. **Knowing why**
   Children must understand the rationale for all of the strategies they learn in therapy, for they cannot meaningfully select which

approach to use in a particular situation if they do not know why the approach works. We can help children develop their understanding of the rationale for therapy techniques by teaching them to think critically and to actively engage in problem-solving activities to determine their own "best practices" in their journeys of dealing with stuttering.

3. **Increasing self-confidence**
A child who stutters must learn to take risks if she wishes to improve her communication skills. A child can only take risks if she has the self-confidence to know that she can handle the outcome. Self-confidence also increases the child's ability to advocate for herself and educate others about stuttering.

4. **Knowing that she is okay even if she stutters**
A child must learn to validate herself and remind herself that it is okay to stutter. Society, and the people in the child's environment, do not always give this message. We can help the child internalize the fact that she is okay by continually demonstrating our own belief in the child's worth and value. As the child becomes more accepting of herself and of her stuttering, her ability to validate herself will increase and, ultimately, she will be able to successfully advocate for herself in many different life situations.

5. **Utilizing resources and support**
Becoming empowered does not mean that the child has to deal with her stuttering entirely on her own. Children and their families can take advantage of numerous resources, such as support groups, literature about stuttering, and allies such as teachers and clinicians to help them learn to face stuttering successfully throughout their lives. As clinicians, we can help children access these resources and develop their support networks by guiding them toward connections that will last a lifetime.

6. **Finding her own voice**
The best speech management tools in the world can only go part of the way to helping a child find her own voice as a speaker and communicator. When a child knows that what she has to say is important enough for her to say it—even if she stutters—then she has learned an important lesson that will help to decrease the impact that stuttering can have on her life.

Although the child who stutters may have many people who want to help her, in the end, there is only so much that speech therapists, teachers, and parents can do. We will not always be with the child as she grows and as she faces new situations throughout her life. Therefore, it is our job to help the child develop the tools she needs to achieve success. These tools include:

- appropriate speech management strategies

- good communication skills

- the ability to advocate for herself and educate others about stuttering

- a strong self-concept

- a sense of empowerment

- problem-solving skills so she can critically evaluate situations she faces

- the courage and self-confidence to put all of these skills into play

If a child is able to develop these skills and maintain them through on-going practice and support, she will be able to get the most out of her life, regardless of whether or not she stutters. This represents the ultimate definition of success in stuttering therapy and the optimal outcome that children and clinicians can work toward.

The example on the next page is written by one of our students. We chose it because it embodies so many of the aspects of change and empowerment that we have discussed throughout this book. In it, Brad, age 15, uses a high school literature assignment to draw parallels between dealing with stuttering and finding his own sense of peace.

My Own Peace by Brad B.

In the book, *A Separate Peace* by John Knowles, the main character, Gene Forrester, eventually finds peace with himself. It is a frustrating and painful experience for Gene. He struggles to understand his relationship with his best friend, Finny. I have a personal situation, which I have had to come to peace with. It has been a long journey for me.

When I was in second grade, I began to talk differently than I had before. I began to have speech disfluency. In other words, I stuttered. This was very difficult for me. It made me feel different from the other kids. I couldn't figure out what was happening to my speech. Some of the other kids started to make fun of me. This was hard to deal with!

As time passed, it seemed like my speech was gradually getting worse. There were times when I couldn't say a sentence without stuttering. Since I was having so much trouble speaking, I didn't even want to raise my hand or speak in class. Sometimes I couldn't even talk to my friends. I remember when it was time to do the lunch count, I couldn't even say "hot" or "cold."

I really wanted to get my speech better, but going to the school speech teacher wasn't helping. Also, it made me feel embarrassed to be taken out of class to see her. My parents found a private speech pathologist who thought she could possibly help me. At first, I was nervous to see her and talk to her. After a while, I became comfortable working with her and talking about my problems with her.

For a long time, I didn't want to admit or accept that I stuttered. I thought that one day I would wake up and no longer stutter. In the meantime, I tried to hide my stuttering as much as possible. I tried to do this by not volunteering in class, or not talking to my friends when I was having a lot of trouble speaking. As it turns out, this was not the best way to handle my problem.

Over the years, I have learned different ways of managing my speech. These are techniques known as "speech tools." I have also learned to face my fears, such as calling people on the phone and giving presentations. Over the past eight years, I have seen dramatic improvement in managing my speech and overcoming my anxiety. There have been many ups and downs along the way, but I am heading in the right direction.

It is a long journey for me. I have learned to accept that I will always stutter. I also know that I should talk whenever I want to communicate. I am slowly learning that stuttering should not control my life. I must control my own life. Maybe some day the medical world will come up with something to help those who stutter, but for now I must be able to accept and live with my stuttering. I will not let stuttering define my life.

Example "I Can . . . Solve Problems"

Name _____ Lisa _____ Grade ___ 3 ___ Date _____

Fill in the blanks with your best thinking and you can come up with your own problem-solving plan. Invite others who may be helpful to complete their own pages.

Name It	The problem is:
	Kids tease me about my stuttering and it makes me mad.

Drain Your Brain

Here are ALL the things I can think of to solve this problem.

Punch somebody.

Tell the teacher.

Ignore them.

Say "Get a life."

Scream <u>really</u> loud!

Give them "the look."

Walk away.

Tease back like "So what, you're ugly."

Say "What's your point?"

Tell my mom.

Tell the playground supervisor.

Do something they don't expect.

Look Ahead

Plug in each idea from "Drain Your Brain" and think more about **what might happen** with each one.

I believe if I _____,

then _____.

Group 'em	Decide which ideas are good for you and which may not be so helpful.

	These could work!	Oops, maybe not. . .
	Tell the teacher. Ignore them. Walk away. Say "What's your point?" Give "the look." Do something they don't expect.	Punching Teasing back Screaming Telling Mom (she might call their parents.)

Pick and Plan	The one I want to try now is: Give "the look" and walk away.

Rate It	Come back and discuss whether the idea you picked was helpful or not. Tell Ms. N. about it next week. This idea did/did not help because:

Do-overs Allowed!	Go back to the drawing board. Ask yourself: • Is the problem listed above *really* the problem, or could it be something else? • Do I need to brainstorm again? • Can others help me brainstorm? • Is there something else from my "These could work!" list that I could try?

About Teasing and Bullying ─────────────

Name _____ Grade _____ Date _____

Complete this page with YOUR ideas about teasing and bullying. Use your best thoughts and be honest in your answers.

I think that teasing and bullying is caused by _____

_____

Everybody gets teased or bullied about something, sometimes.   True   False

People usually tease because _____

_____

I have seen (or heard) kids get teased about _____

_____

Teasers and bullies have a lot of friends.   True   False

People who tease or bully are _____

Bullies should have to _____

Getting teased can make someone feel _____

One time, I got teased about _____

It made me feel _____

When it happened, I (what did you do/say?) _____

_____

Fighting usually solves problems.   True   False

One time I teased someone about _____

Some kids react to bullying by:

_____ walking away   _____ telling their parents

_____ fighting or pushing   _____ telling their teachers

_____ name calling   _____ saying "stop it"

_____ yelling   _____ crying

_____ ignoring the bully completely

Some things I have tried before are _____

I think some good ways to handle teasing and bullying are _____

_____

Teacher Training Module _____

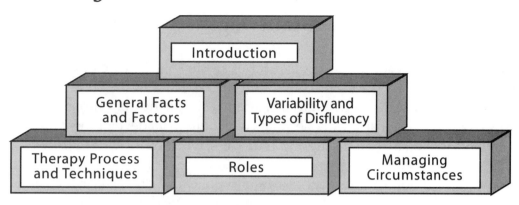

This year, you have a child who stutters in your classroom.

As the SLP working with _____, I am available as your resource person to provide you with information and support regarding stuttering.

During the next week, I will send you a short informational handout each day to provide you with some of the basic information about stuttering so you will be able to support your student in the classroom. (See topics above.)

Of course, we will also discuss the individual child at other times so we can to collaborate regarding specifics of his or her situation.

For a child who stutters, it is important for everyone in the environment to develop and maintain a "team" atmosphere so we can support him or her through the changes that take place over time. You, as the educator, are an *essential* part of this team. Other team members will include parents and significant others (e.g., peers, family members). As part of the support team, I will be available to you to discuss and problem solve any situations or questions that arise while the child is in your classroom.

Please read each handout, and feel free to make comments or ask questions about any of the information. The best time to reach me is _____ at _____. However, I can be flexible so that we may meet or talk at your convenience.

Thank you for your cooperation in this child's progress.

Sincerely,

_____
Speech-Language Pathologist

Day 1: General Facts About Stuttering

There are many myths surrounding the disorder of stuttering. They can be attributed to the lack of understanding of this disorder throughout history, and to the continuing attempts to explain stuttering in simplistic ways. Stuttering defies simplistic definitions and explanations. It is a complex disorder with many variables that contribute to its development and maintenance. Below are a few of the facts about stuttering that are important for you to understand.

- Even though we don't have exact answers to the cause of stuttering, current research suggests that there are several factors involved, including factors inherent to the child and those involving environment.

- Stuttering is not caused by past psychological or physical trauma.

- Stuttering is not linked to intelligence. Children who stutter do not have lower intelligence than their peers because they stutter. Just as each *child* is different, each child who stutters is different. Stuttering occurs in children with gifted intelligences as well as those who struggle with learning.

- Studies have demonstrated that approximately 1% of the population stutters. Current estimates are that about three million Americans stutter. The ratio of males to females who stutter has been reported to be approximately 3:1 or more.

- Many children who exhibit beginning signs of stuttering in preschool years do develop through their disfluencies. Unfortunately, however, we cannot predict which preschool children will recover and which children will develop a lifelong stuttering condition. Therefore, early assessment, diagnosis and treatment are strongly recommended.

- There are no cures or "quick fixes" for stuttering. Speech therapy can help a person who stutters manage speech and make long-term changes over time.

Causal vs. Precipitating Factors

Developmental stuttering most likely occurs between the ages of two and five years. This seems to coincide with the rapid expansion of speech and language skills during these formative years of a child's development.

The variables that contribute to the maintenance of the disorder in some individuals include neurophysiological, social, psychological, cognitive, and linguistic factors. Because of the number of variables that affect stuttering, it is seen as a highly complex disorder.

Current studies suggest that stuttering can be decreased by making changes in speech patterns or decreasing the demands on the speech-motor and language systems. This finding has implications for treatment for it suggests that adjustments to speech behaviors, modifications to the environment, and the development of coping strategies are all part of the process of therapy. We will be discussing some of the treatment factors in the handouts that follow each day.

When Speaking with Someone Who Stutters

In general, the following responses are appropriate when speaking with anyone who stutters:

Do not finish. Allow the child to get the message completed. Reflect what you have heard so that the child knows you have understood him or her, and he or she is given an opportunity to repair the message, if necessary.

Do not rush. Time pressure can be a problem for many children who stutter. When listeners inadvertently or purposefully put time limits on communication, children who stutter may feel a need to speak quickly. This can build tension in speech muscles, thereby causing increased stuttering.

Maintain relaxed body language. Maintain normal eye contact and be aware of head nodding or gestures that may rush a child to complete a message.

Do not give advice. Suggestions such as "slow down," "take a deep breath," "start over," and "think about what you are going to say," may be well-meaning and *seemingly* helpful for a child who is struggling with communication. In fact, these suggestions can create unnecessary pressure on the child. As listeners, we need to wait patiently and continue to encourage communication no matter how it is presented: fluently or with stuttering.

Day 2: Variability/Cyclic Nature of Stuttering

One question we are often asked is: "Why is this child relatively fluent on some days and struggling more on others?"

The short answer to this question is that stuttering is, by nature, a cyclic and variable disorder. These "good days and bad days" add to the mystery surrounding stuttering to those who don't understand the complexity of the variables that can affect the cycles of stuttering (see Day 1).

It is important to understand that there are many interpersonal and environmental factors that may disrupt fluency in some children. *Some example factors are listed below. Not all factors are listed, and not all of those listed are universally disruptive to all children who stutter.*

loss of listener attention	high, self-imposed expectations
interruptions	excitement
time pressure	word retrieval difficulties
demand speech	sensitivity
rapid speech models	complexity of language/vocabulary
fatigue	unexpected events
competitive situations	

Types of Disfluency

Listed below are types of disfluency and stuttering behaviors that you may observe in the speech of the child in your classroom. As you are an integral part of this child's therapy progress, these are important distinctions of which you should be aware. This understanding will help you use your observational skills to provide feedback on progress from your perspective as the classroom educator.

"Normal" Disfluencies

These are types of "breaks" in speech fluency that many speakers experience.

hesitations	silence during or between messages
revisions	starting a message, stopping, and starting over again (I want - I need that.")
interjections	"um," "like," "you know"
word repetitions	"I-I want you to go."
phrase repetitions	"and then, and then"

"Stuttered" Disfluencies

whole word repetitions	"We - We - We - We are going home."
syllable repetitions	"Can I ta-take this one?"
sound repetitions	"That is m - m - m - my book."
prolongations	"Please sssssssend it in the mail."
blocks	Excessive tension when trying to speak and no sound comes forth (seems as though the word gets "stuck")

Other behaviors that MAY be a part of the repertoire of the child who stutters in your classroom:

extra verbalizations	emitting sounds that seem to "start" other words
facial movements	eye blinking, facial tension, etc.
bodily tension	head nodding, arm movements, etc.
avoidance behaviors	word substitutions, avoiding speaking, etc.

Understanding Secondary Behaviors

Not all children who stutter experience visibly increased tension or extraneous movements in their bodies. It is important to know that these types of behaviors can come from the child's feeling of loss of control over the speech mechanism. When a child who stutters increases tension or "pushes" to get the word out, he or she can begin to push harder and harder, thus building tension in facial or other muscles of his or her body. When a child begins to gain control of the "speech machine" through relaxation and speech therapy techniques, these secondary behaviors tend to fade away, as their reason for being is no longer necessary.

Avoidance Behaviors

Not all children who stutter avoid, but it is important for you to understand *how to spot* it if it occurs. Some children use many "tricks" to avoid stuttering. Avoidance behaviors can manifest themselves in many ways. Some examples include changing the word they are going to say, pretending to be confused when called upon to read or answer questions, saying "I don't know" even when they *do* know the answer, leaving the class to go to the bathroom, never volunteering to read or answer questions, allowing others to answer for them in group activities, etc. By knowing some of these possibilities and being the "eyes" for the SLP, you can help to make important therapy decisions that will benefit the child's overall success in therapy.

Day 3:   The Therapy Process

"What Happens in the Speech Room?"

Understanding the Process: Speech therapy is not a *cure* for stuttering. There are no instant cures. Therapy is a *process* of change *over time*.

Goals and Balance: It is important to understand that the ultimate goal of school-age stuttering therapy for a child who has established patterns of stuttering behaviors is NOT perfectly fluent speech. It is *effective communication*. We are providing therapy within a *balance* of changing speech behaviors and improving attitudes about speech and self.

Speech Strategies and How We Use Them

Occasionally, you may be invited to therapy sessions so you can learn what children who stutter do in therapy. In these sessions, the child may teach you some of the strategies so you will be able to recognize when he or she is using them in the classroom. Following is a brief overview of some of the strategies he or she *may* be learning over time.

Learning how to talk more easily involves decreasing and controlling the amount of tension in the speech muscles. In order to help children speak more fluently, we teach them various tools, such as:

- The Speech Machine: discovering what structures are involved in the production of speech, and how these structures must work together for the machine to work efficiently

- Easy Starts: learning to "turn on" the speech machine in a gradual, easy way

- Pausing/Phrasing: allowing time between phrases in structured and conversational speech (in order to relax tension in speech muscles or to use speech techniques, etc.)

Sometimes, "easy speech" tools aren't enough to provide sufficient support for increasing fluency and ease of communication. Therefore, we also have a set of tools the child can use when he or she is already experiencing a moment of stuttering which is designed to gain control of the tension in speech muscles.

- Location of Tension: discovering where tension can occur in speech muscles

- Pull Outs/Slide Outs: easing out of tension during moments of stuttering

- Block-Outs: feeling a moment of tension, stopping, releasing the tension, and starting over with an easy start or easier stutter

- Cancellations: going back to "take control" of a previously stuttered word by releasing tension and approaching the word again in a less tense way

- Voluntary Stuttering: using short, easy, purposeful stuttering behaviors to desensitize a child to moments of stuttering

As discussed earlier, we will also be paying attention to and working with *attitudes about speech and self.* Other issues may also arise over time (e.g., teasing, responsibility, motivation, self-esteem), and you may be asked to participate in problem-solving or brainstorming discussions to identify ways to help the child deal with the situations he or she faces because of his or her stuttering.

Day 4: Roles

Everyone in the environment of the child who stutters will have roles in the process of therapy. My role as SLP includes providing speech therapy services, initiating and maintaining consultative efforts, and acting as a liaison among parents, administrators, and educators. Above all, I am your source of information and support about stuttering.

Below are listed some of the roles that educators can play in the lives of children who stutter.

What you can do: **You are a model! You not only set the *learning* atmosphere in your classroom, you set the *communicative* atmosphere, as well.**

1. Provide a comfortable communication environment by:

   - minimizing interruptions
   - modeling thinking time (e.g., "Let me think about that. Yes, I will agree on that point.")
   - allowing increased response time (decrease time pressure)
   - reflecting the messages that your students send

   These communicative strategies help to set the atmosphere that *what* a person is saying (the message) is much more important than *how* he or she says it (the delivery).

2. Exhibit positive attitudes regarding communication.

   The ideal model demonstrates patience and acceptance. By creating an atmosphere where differences between children are accepted, it is possible to provide support for the child who stutters, as well as all other children in the classroom. Patient speaking (interaction) and listening (reflection) styles can be models for children to experience the concept that everyone gets time for thinking, listening, and responding. These types of communicative models can serve to enhance fluency goals as well as to decrease the overall stress in the environment of your classroom.

3. Be an observer.

   You are the liaison between therapy and the classroom. Along with being able to provide feedback regarding types of stuttering that you see, you are also in a unique position to observe situations that seem to either promote fluency *or* exacerbate stuttering. By observing and reporting situations, you are providing an invaluable perspective that will help to set appropriate goals for the child in your classroom.

4. Be a source of understanding and support.

   You are in the position to help the child accept himself or herself. By viewing the child as a *whole* child and not focusing on his or her stuttering behaviors, your responses and reactions can send the message that his or her ideas are an important addition to the overall environment of the classroom.

When you instill confidence and provide opportunities for success in speaking situations in the classroom, you can create and maintain part of the support structure that is the foundation for long-term success.

With my guidance, you can also provide opportunities for private discussions about speech and stuttering. These can be matter-of-fact discussions about classroom situations. The child can help you understand his or her wishes and plans regarding his or her expectations for the classroom or ability to participate in classroom communications.

And finally, by recognizing successes and strengths rather than focusing (or allowing the child to focus) on perceived weakness, you can begin to increase this child's confidence and self-esteem in everyday academic situations.

5. Monitor the messages that you send.

The "Whole Child"
Stuttering is something that this child *does*, not something that he or she *is*. It is important to see the "whole child" in the process. The child may like animals, enjoy video games, and have an artistic side that needs to be tapped into. Or the child may like basketball, play the saxophone, and be an avid reader. All of these things are what we need to discover in order to know *the child*. Stuttering is simply a small part of the whole child in your classroom.

Expectations for Fluency
In general, send and model the message that "Mistakes are okay. They are opportunities for learning" is extremely helpful for children who stutter (and all children for that matter). Specifically, it is important to send the message that "stuttering is okay; you have good ideas that I want to hear, no matter how they are presented."

Why Doesn't the Child Just Use His or Her Tools?

This is a common question that speaks to the expectations that arise when a child has been in therapy for a while. It is important to consider that children learn and use tools at different rates. They may also go through periods of time when speech tools may simply not be a priority for them. Remember, when some children use speech tools, they are changing the way they are talking almost every time they open their mouths! Think about how difficult this must be. It is possible to liken this task to asking you to now change your way of walking (say, walking backward) every time you attempt to do so from now on. Try to remember to do *that* for even one day! We must be patient and send the message that we understand the challenges that the child is facing, and that we are there to support him or her no matter what!

Day 5:   Managing Circumstances

In the classroom, you will encounter situations in which you may feel unsure of appropriate responses. In this section, you will find general suggestions for some of these circumstances. Once again, *the team (including the child) needs to be a part of the decisions about whether or how to use these strategies.* Thus, these are just examples of ideas that may be helpful. Please use your own knowledge of the child and your experience as an educator to guide you in the decision-making process regarding the "best course of action."

Everyday Occurrences

1. Classroom discussions can be handled by allowing increased response time and encouraging everyone to contribute to the exchange of ideas.

2. Reading aloud is a situation that may increase anxiety if the child who stutters must wait for his or her turn. To minimize this, you may wish to consider randomly choosing students.

3. During group interactions, one must monitor the amount of collaboration that is occurring and, when possible, pair the child who stutters with easy-going, patient partners who allow him or her to contribute equally.

4. When it is time for answering questions, you can help by not rewarding quick call-out answers (e.g., "Around the World" types of games). Taking turns, modeling thinking time, and random selection are helpful strategies in this type of situation.

Special Situations

1. Classroom presentations may pose problems for children who stutter (and many other children in your classroom!). It is important to approach these presentations in a matter-of-fact way, and to develop a plan with the team members that support the needs of the child. Flexibility will be necessary at times regarding the method of presentation. It is during these times that your ability to demonstrate flexibility and your willingness to problem solve with the child will be most important. When giving a grade for the oral report, content may be considered the most important factor in the final grade.

2. "How do I handle questions from peers?" This is a frequently asked question. Once again, team members are the answer. Collaborate with those who know the child (e.g., parent, educators, the child) for input if this situation arises. The best answers can only come from the child himself or from those who know the child best. When it is time, children who stutter can be guided and empowered to field questions about stuttering on their own.

Rule of thumb: Demonstrate respect for differences in a matter-of-fact manner. You can show children that "we all have something new we are learning about."

3. Teasing is a part of everyday life for children at one time or another and for one reason or another. An environment of acceptance of differences can go a long way toward decreasing episodes of teasing among your students. Unfortunately, we cannot eliminate teasing and bullying altogether. Therefore, we must be prepared to respond appropriately to episodes of teasing involving the child who stutters. We must also be prepared to empower the child who stutters with strategies for dealing with teasing on his or her own. The goal of these strategies must always be to best respond (instead of react) to teasing in ways that continue to support the child's self esteem and confidence.

Example strategies:

- Increasing understanding and respect for differences
- Developing an atmosphere of zero tolerance for intolerance
- If mimicking or teasing are persistent, direct intervention may be warranted in a firm but polite and diplomatic manner. We must then be diligent in following up to make certain our intervention has not caused retributions for the child who stutters.
- Once again, *problem solving* with the child who stutters and other team members may bring about the best ideas for plans of action when dealing with teasing.

In children's literature, there are many books about teasing and bullying. Using these resources, as well as turning to experts that may be available in your district (e.g., social worker, psychologist) can be helpful developing a variety of strategies for dealing with teasing.

I hope the information shared over the past few days has been helpful. If you need further information, please don't hesitate to contact me.

Phone _____   Best time to call _____

E-mail _____

Speech-Language Pathologist _____

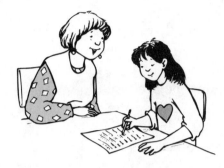

At the beginning of this book, we highlighted the fact that many practicing clinicians do not feel comfortable working with school-age children who stutter. Our primary objectives in writing this book were to help clinicians enhance their knowledge about the stuttering disorder, expand their appreciation for the child's experience of stuttering, and increase their confidence in their own skills for working with stuttering. In this way, we sought to improve clinicians' ability to help children who stutter and increase their success in treatment.

Planning for Success

We sought to accomplish our goals by first emphasizing the importance of taking a broad-based view of the stuttering disorder. *Stuttering is more than just a behavior*—it is a communication disorder that can affect every aspect of a child's life. Thus, when approaching the diagnosis and treatment of stuttering in school-age children, you need to think about the speech behaviors *in addition to* the child's reactions to stuttering, the overall impact of stuttering on the child's ability to communicate in daily situations, and the reactions of the people in the child's environment. Unless you address the full impact of a child's stuttering disorder, your treatment will be incomplete and your success will be limited.

We also highlighted several other aspects of the stuttering disorder that affect our clinical practice. For example, it is important for clinicians, children who stutter, and everybody in the children's environment to realize that *stuttering is variable*. The behaviors and reactions seen in one situation are not necessarily the same as those seen in another situation. In addition, *different children stutter in different ways*, so every child needs an individualized treatment program that is specifically tailored to address his individual concerns. Together, these two facts have significant implications for the diagnostic process, for they mean that you must examine many different aspects of a child's experience to determine whether treatment is indicated and to define what the nature of that treatment should be. Furthermore, the individual variability of stuttering means that you should not attempt to apply a "canned" treatment approach to all children who stutter, for if you do, your intervention will not be able to address the full complexity of each child's individual experiences with stuttering. *Individualized therapy is critical to success.*

Of course, there is a certain consistency to the therapy programs we develop for school-age children who stutter. For those children who have needs in the area of improving speech fluency, we teach a variety of strategies designed to *modify the timing and tension* of speech production (e.g., easy starts, light contacts, changes to communication rate, pausing). Those same children may also need to reduce the severity of their stuttering events, so we also teach strategies for *reducing physical tension* during stuttering such as cancellation or block-outs, easing out or slide outs, and easy stuttering. For those children who need to *reduce their negative affective, behavioral, or cognitive reactions* to stuttering, we focus on desensitization, voluntary stuttering or pseudo-stuttering, and self-disclosure. To facilitate generalization and *reduce the negative consequences of stuttering* for the child's life overall, we focus on ensuring that the child has practiced every strategy and goal in every situation he faces (working along a hierarchy from easier to harder situations). We also work to ensure that the child can *say anything and do anything regardless of the fact that he stutters*. Finally we want to ensure that everybody in the child's environment understands and accepts the goals of treatment. We help the child learn how to teach others about his speech, and we help him learn how to *explain his therapy goals, procedures, and successes* to parents, teachers, and peers. This will help him develop the tools he will need so he can *advocate for himself* throughout his life.

Throughout this book, we have underscored the importance of adopting a definition of success that allows for the fact that the child is quite likely to continue stuttering in some fashion even at the conclusion of formal therapy. Rather than focusing on a (largely unattainable) goal of "perfect" or "normal" fluency, we seek to help the child learn to *communicate effectively* with increased fluency, decreased tension, reduced negative reactions, minimal impact of stuttering, and an environment that is both supportive and accepting. *This* is the definition of true success, and this is a goal that school-age children who stutter (and their clinicians) can realistically hope to achieve.

Children Who Stutter Are on a Journey

Earlier in this book, we pointed out that children who stutter are each on a journey. Remember that the end point of their journeys are not an arbitrary, predefined level of fluency or the completion of a programmed treatment approach. Instead, the purpose of their journeys is to help them become *the best possible* communicators *they can be*. Along the way, they will have to take risks so they can face their fears about stuttering, learn new ways of talking, and increase their abilities to speak effectively. The tasks they have before them are not easy but with your help, they can do it.

By working with children who stutter to help them approach, explore, understand, and change their stuttering, you can be their partner in their journeys—for a time. Keep in mind, though, that their journeys will continue long after they have finished working with you. Their journeys will carry them throughout their lives, into many new situations and many new challenges. Therefore, your goal in therapy should not simply be to "get them fluent" when they are with you, or even just while they are in school. Instead, your goal should be to help them learn the skills they will need to manage their speech and their stuttering over the long term. By focusing on the big picture and long-term success, you will be able to give children the tools they really need to achieve their greatest success, both in and out of therapy, both in the short term and throughout their lives.

You Are on a Journey Too

As an SLP, your clinical skills are always developing and always expanding. You, too, are on a journey. Your goal is to become the best clinician you can be. As you continue the process of developing your skills for helping children who stutter, we hope you remember that the many ways of treating stuttering is similar to treating other disorders within your scope of practice. So many of the skills and strategies used for helping children with articulation, language, or other communication disorders apply directly to the process of helping children who stutter. You can draw upon your many existing skills to provide an excellent foundation for developing your skills to help children who stutter.

We also hope that you will take the opportunity to expand your knowledge and understanding about stuttering. One way you can work toward this important goal is to be willing to take a risk and *enter the world of the child who stutters*. Spend time trying to understand his communication experiences, including the tension and struggle, the emotional reactions and fear, and the negative consequences that may occur. Talk with adults who stutter and the family members of children who stutter by participating in stuttering support groups so you can understand the overall life impact of stuttering. Experiment with different ways of stuttering and different ways of changing stuttering so you can understand what you are asking your young students to do in therapy while appreciating the challenges your students may face.

Through these and other exercises, you can develop a greater appreciation for the child's experience of stuttering, and this will further increase your comfort with stuttering and enhance your ability to provide excellent therapy for young children who stutter.

You Can Do It!

We hope this book has helped you approach the task of working with school-age children who stutter with a greater sense of comfort and confidence in yourself. Above all, we want you to remember that it *is* possible for you to become an excellent stuttering therapist. Trust yourself and your clinical skills, draw upon available resources, and continue to push yourself to take risks and explore new approaches. Soon, you will find that you *can* do it—you *can* approach the problem of childhood stuttering with the knowledge that that you *will* be able to help your young students learn to communicate more effectively and overcome the challenges of stuttering in their lives.

Adams, M.R. (1980). The young stutterer: Diagnosis, treatment and assessment of progress. *Seminars in Speech, Language and Hearing, 1,* 289-299.

Ambrose, N. & Yairi, E. (1999). Normative disfluency data for early childhood stuttering. *Journal of Speech, Language, & Hearing Research, 42,* 895-909.

Ambrose, N., Yairi, E., & Cox, N. (1993). Genetic aspects of early childhood stuttering. *Journal of Speech and Hearing Research, 36,* 701-706.

American Speech-Language-Hearing Association. (2003). Code of ethics (revised). *ASHA Supplement, 23,* 13-15.

Andrews, G. & Harris, M. (1964). The syndrome of stuttering. *Clinics in Developmental Medicine,* 17. London: Spastics Society Medical Education and Information Unit, in association with Wm. Heinemann Medical Books.

Andrews, J. & Andrews, M. (2000). *Family-based treatment in communicative disorders: A systematic approach* (2nd ed.). DeKalb, IL: Janelle Publications, Inc.

Battle, D. (1998). *Communication disorders in multicultural populations* (2nd ed.). Butterworth-Heinemann: Boston, MA.

Bernstein Ratner, N. (1995). Treating the child with concomitant grammatical or phonological impairment. *Language, Speech, and Hearing Services in Schools, 2,* 180-186.

Bernstein Ratner, N. (1997). Stuttering: A Psycholinguistic Perspective. In R. Curlee & G. Siegel (Eds.), *Nature and treatment of stuttering: New directions* (2nd ed., pp. 97-127). Needham Heights, MA: Allyn & Bacon.

Bernstein Ratner, N.E. (1993). Parents, children, and stuttering. *Seminars in Speech and Language, 14(3),* 238-247.

Bernstein Ratner, N.E. (1997). Leaving Las Vegas: Clinical odds and individual outcomes. *American Journal of Speech-Language Pathology, 6(2),* 29-33.

Bloodstein, O. (1984). Stuttering as an anticipatory struggle disorder. In R.F. Curlee & W. Perkins (Eds.), *Nature and treatment of stuttering: New directions,* (pp. 171-186). Needham Heights, MA: Allyn & Bacon.

Bloodstein, O. (1993). *Stuttering: The Search for a Cause and Cure.* Needham Heights, MA: Allyn & Bacon.

Bloodstein, O. (1995). *A handbook on stuttering* (5th ed.). San Diego, CA: Singular Publishing Group.

Bloom, C.M. & Cooperman, D.K. (1999). *Synergistic stuttering therapy: A holistic approach.* Boston: Butterworth-Heinemann.

Bothe, A. (2002). Speech modification approaches to stuttering treatment in schools. *Seminars in Speech and Language, 23*, 181-186.

Bradberry, A. (1997). The role of support groups and stuttering therapy. *Seminars in Speech and Language, 18*, 391-399.

Bradberry, A. & Reardon, N. (1999). *Our voices: Inspirational insights from young people who stutter.* Anaheim Hills, CA: National Stuttering Association.

Breitenfeldt, D.H. & Lorenz, D.R. (2000). *Successful stuttering management program (SSMP): For Adolescent and Adult Stutterers* (2nd ed.). Cheney, WA: Eastern Washington University.

Callaghan, S. & Joseph, S. (1995). Self-concept and peer victimization among school children. *Personality & Individual Differences, 18*, 161-163.

Campbell, J. (2003). Therapy for elementary school-age children who stutter. In H. Gregory (Ed.), *Stuttering Therapy Rationale and Procedures,* (pp. 217-262). Boston: Allyn & Bacon.

Campbell, J. & Hill, D. (1987). *Systematic disfluency analysis: Accountability for differential evaluation and treatment.* Miniseminar presented to the Annual Convention of the American Speech-Language-Hearing Association. New Orleans, LA.

Chmela, K. & Reardon, N. (2001). *The school-age child who stutters: working effectively with attitudes and emotions.* Memphis, TN: Stuttering Foundation of America.

Conture, E.G. (2001). *Stuttering: Its Nature, Diagnosis, and Treatment.* Needham Heights, MA: Allyn & Bacon.

Conture, E.G. & Guitar, B. (1993). Evaluating efficacy of treatment of stuttering: School-age children. *Journal of Fluency Disorders, 18*, 253-287.

Conture, E.G., Louko, L.J., & Edwards, M.L. (1993). Simultaneously treating stuttering and disordered phonology in children: Experimental therapy, preliminary findings. *American Journal of Speech-Language-Pathology, 2 (3)*, 72-81.

Cooper, E.B. (1986). Treatment of disfluency: future trends. *Journal of Fluency Disorders, 11*, 317-327.

Cordes, A.K. (1994). The reliability of observational data: I. Theories and methods of speech-language pathology. *Journal of Speech and Hearing Research, 37*, 264-278.

Cordes, A.K. (1998). Current status of the stuttering treatment literature. In A.K. Cordes & R.J. Ingham (Eds.), *Toward treatment efficacy in stuttering: A search for empirical bases,* (pp. 113-144). Austin, TX: Pro-Ed.

Cordes, A.K. & Ingham, R.J. (1994a). The reliability of observational data: II. Issues in the identification and measurement of stuttering events. *Journal of Speech and Hearing Research, 37*, 279-294.

Cordes, A.K. & Ingham, R.J. (1994b). Time-interval measurement of stuttering: Effects of interval duration. *Journal of Speech and Hearing Research, 37,* 779-788.

Cordes, A.K. & Ingham, R.J. (1995). Judgments of stuttered and nonstuttered intervals by recognized authorities in stuttering research. *Journal of Speech and Hearing Research, 38,* 33-41.

Costello, J.M. & Hurst, M.R. (1981). An analysis of the relationship among stuttering behaviors. *Journal of Speech and Hearing Research, 24,* 247-256.

Costello, J.M. & Ingham, R.J. (1984). Assessment strategies for stuttering. In R.F. Curlee & W.H. Perkins (Eds.). *Nature and treatment of stuttering: New directions.* San Diego: College-Hill Press.

Crowe, T. (1997). *Applications of counseling in speech language pathology and audiology.* Baltimore: Williams and Wilkins.

Curlee, R.F. (1993). Identification and management of beginning stuttering. In R.F. Curlee (Ed.). *Stuttering and related disorders of fluency.* (1-22). New York: Thieme Medical Publishers.

Curlee, R.F. (Ed.) (1999). *Stuttering and Related Disorders of Fluency* (2nd ed.) New York: Thieme Publishers.

Curlee, R. & Siegel, G. (Eds.) (1997). *Nature and treatment of stuttering: New directions* (2nd ed.). Needham Heights, MA: Allyn & Bacon.

Curlee, R.F. & Yairi, E. (1997). Early intervention with early childhood stuttering: A critical examination of the data. *American Journal of Speech-Language Pathology, 6 (2),* 8-18.

deGeus, E. (2001). *Sometime I just stutter: A book for children between the ages of 7 and 12.* Memphis, TN: Stuttering Foundation of America.

Dell, C. (1993). Treating school-age stutterers. In R. Curlee (Ed.). *Stuttering and related disorders of fluency.* New York: Thieme Medical Publishers.

DeNil, L.F. & Brutten, G.J. (1991). Speech-associated attitudes of stuttering and nonstuttering children. *Journal of Speech and Hearing Research, 34,* 60-66.

Egan, G. (2002). *The Skilled Helper* (7th ed.). Pacific Grove, CA: Brooks/Cole Publishers.

Faber, A. & Mazlish, E. (1999). *How to talk so kids will listen and listen so kids will talk* (20th Anniversary ed.). New York: Avon Books.

Finn, P. (2003). Self-regulation and the management of stuttering. *Seminars in Speech and Language, 24,* 27-32.

Fosnot, S.M. (1993). Research design for examining treatment efficacy in fluency disorders. *Journal of Fluency Disorders, 18,* 221-251.

Freedman, J. (2002). *Easing the teasing: How parents can help their kids cope*. Chicago: Contemporary McGraw-Hill.

Gillespie S. & Cooper E. (1973). Prevalence of speech problems in junior and senior high schools. *Journal of Speech and Hearing Research, 34,* 739-743.

Gilman, M. & Yaruss, J.S. (2000). Relaxation and somatic education in stuttering treatment. *Journal of Fluency Disorders, 25,* 59-76.

Gordon, P.A. & Luper, H.L. (1992a). The early identification of beginning stuttering I: Protocols. *American Journal of Speech-Language Pathology: A Journal of Clinical Practice, 1(3),* 43-53.

Gordon, P.A. & Luper, H.L. (1992b). The early identification of beginning stuttering II: Problems. *American Journal of Speech-Language Pathology: A Journal of Clinical Practice, 1(4),* 49-55.

Gottwald, S. & Hall, N. (2002). Stuttering treatment in schools: Developing family and teacher partnerships. *Seminars in Speech and Language, 23,* 41-46.

Gregory, H.H. (Ed.). (1979). *Controversies about stuttering therapy*. Baltimore, MD: University Park Press.

Gregory, H.H. (1995). Analysis and commentary. *Language, Speech, and Hearing Services in Schools, 26,* 196-200.

Gregory, H.H. (2003). *Stuttering therapy: Rationale and procedures*. Boston, MA: Allyn & Bacon.

Gregory, H.H. & Hill, D. (1999). Differential evaluation-differential treatment for stuttering children. In R.F. Curlee (Ed.), *Stuttering and related disorders of fluency* (2nd ed, pp. 22-42). New York: Thieme Medical Publishers.

Guitar, B. (1998). *Stuttering: An integrated approach to its nature and treatment*. (2nd ed.). Baltimore, MD: Williams & Wilkins.

Hall, P.K. (1977). The occurrence of disfluencies in language-disordered school-age children. *Journal of Speech and Hearing Disorders, 42,* 364-369.

Harris, V., Onslow, M., Packman, A., Harrison, E., & Menzies R. (2002). An experimental investigation of the impact of the Lidcombe Program on early stuttering. *Journal of Fluency Disorders, 27,* 203-213.

Ingham, J.C. (1999). Behavioral treatment of young children who stutter: An extended length of utterance method. In R.F. Curlee (Ed.), *Stuttering and Related Disorders of Fluency* (2nd ed., pp. 80-109). New York: Thieme Publishers.

Ingham, R.J. (1984). *Stuttering and behavior therapy: Current status and experimental foundations*. San Diego, CA: College-Hill Press.

Ingham, R.J. & Cordes, A.K. (1997). Self-measurement and evaluating stuttering treatment efficacy. In R.F. Curlee & G.M. Siegel (Eds.), *Nature and treatment of stuttering: New directions* (2nd ed., pp. 413-437). Needham Heights: MA: Allyn & Bacon.

Ingham, R.J. & Onslow, M. (1985). Measurement and modification of speech naturalness during stuttering therapy. *Journal of Speech and Hearing Disorders, 50*, 261-281.

Jacobson, E. (1938). *Progressive relaxation* (2nd ed.). Chicago: The University of Chicago Press.

Johnson, W. (1949). An open letter to the mother of a "stuttering" child. *Journal of Speech and Hearing Disorders, 14*, 3-8.

Johnson, W. (1961). *Stuttering and What You Can Do About It*. Minneapolis: University of Minnesota Press.

Johnson, W. & Associates (1959). *The Onset of Stuttering*. Minneapolis: University of Minnesota Press.

Johnson, W., Darley, F.L., & Spriestersbach, D.C. (1963). *Diagnostic methods in speech pathology*. New York: Harper & Row.

Kelly, E.M. & Conture, E.G. (1992). Speaking rates, response time latencies, and interrupting behaviors of young stutterers, nonstutterers, and their mothers. *Journal of Speech and Hearing Research, 35*, 1256-1267.

Langevin, M. (1997). Peer teasing project. In E. Healey and H. F. M. Peters (Eds.), *Second World Congress on Fluency Disorders: Proceedings* (pp. 169-171). The Netherlands: Nijmegen University Press.

Lass, N., Ruscello, D., Schmitt, J., Pannbacker, M., Orlando, M., Dean, K., Ruziska, J., & Bradshaw, K. (1992) Teachers' perceptions of stutterers. *Language, Speech and Hearing Services in Schools, 23*, 78-81.

Lears, L. (2000). *Ben has something to say: A story about stuttering*. Morton Grove, IL: Albert Whitman & Co.

Leavitt, R. (1974). *The Puerto Ricans: Cultural change and language deviance*. University of Arizona Press: Tucson, AZ.

Lincoln, M. & Harrison, E. (1999). The Lidcombe program. In M. Onslow & A. Packman (Eds.), *The handbook of early stuttering intervention* (pp. 103-118). San Diego, CA: Singular Publishing Group.

Logan, K.J. & LaSalle, L.R. (2003). Developing intervention programs for children with stuttering and concomitant impairments. *Seminars in Speech and Language, 24*, 13-19.

Logan, K.J. & Yaruss, J.S. (1999). Helping parents address attitudinal and emotional factors with young children who stutter. *Contemporary Issues in Communication Science and Disorders, 26*, 69-81.

Louko, L.J., Edwards, M.L., & Conture, E.G. (1990). Phonological characteristics of young stutterers and their normally fluent peers: Preliminary observations. *Journal of Fluency Disorders, 15*, 191-210.

Manning, W. (1999). Progress under the surface and over time. In N. Bernstein Ratner, & E.C. Healey (Eds.), *Stuttering research and practice: Bridging the gap.* (123-130). Mahwah, NJ: Lawrence Erlbaum.

Manning, W. (2001). *Clinical Decision Making in Fluency Disorders* (2nd ed.). San Diego, CA: Singular/Thompson Learning.

Murphy, W. (1999). A preliminary look at shame, guilt, and stuttering. In N. Bernstein Ratner, & E.C. Healey (Eds.), *Stuttering research and practice: Bridging the gap* (pp. 131-142). Mahwah, NJ: Lawrence Erlbaum.

Murphy, W. (1989). *The school-aged child who stutters: dealing effectively with shame and guilt.* Videotape No. 86. Memphis, TN: Stuttering Foundation of America.

Murphy, W. & Quesal, R.W. (2002). Strategies for addressing bullying with the school-age child who stutters. *Seminars in Speech and Language, 23*, 205-211.

Murphy, W. & Reardon, N. (2001). *A classroom presentation about stuttering.* Anaheim, CA: National Stuttering Association.

Neary, A. & Joseph, S. (1994). Peer victimization and its relationship to self-concept and depression among school girls. *Personality & Individual Differences, 16*, 183-186.

Nippold, M. & Rudzinski, M. (1995). Parents' speech and children's stuttering: a critique of the literature. *Journal of Speech, Language, and Hearing Research, 38*, 978-989.

Olson, E. & Bohlman, P. (2002). IDEA '97 and children who stutter: Evaluation and intervention that lead to successful, productive lives. *Seminars in Speech and Language, 23*, 159-164.

Onslow, M. (1996). *Behavior management of stuttering.* San Diego, CA: Singular Publishing Group.

Perkins, W.H. (1990). What is stuttering? *Journal of Speech and Hearing Disorders, 55*, 379-382.

Power, M. (2002). Research-Based Stuttering Therapy. *Perspectives on Fluency Disorder, 12 (1)*, 4-5.

Quesal, R.W. & Yaruss, J.S. (2000). Historical perspectives on stuttering treatment: Dean Williams. *Contemporary Issues in Communication Science and Disorders, 27*, 178-187.

Ramig, P. (1993). The impact of self-help groups on persons who stutter: A call for research. *Journal of Fluency Disorders, 18*, 351-361.

Ramig, P. & Bennett, E. (1997). Clinical management of children: Direct management strategies. In R. Curlee & G. Siegel (Eds.), *Nature and Treatment of Stuttering: New Directions* (2nd ed., pp. 292-312). Needham Heights, MA: Allyn & Bacon.

Reardon, N. & Reeves, L. (2002). Stuttering therapy in partnership with support groups: The best of both worlds. *Seminars in Speech and Language, 23*, 213-218.

Reardon, N. & Yaruss, J.S. (2002). Successful speech therapy in the schools: It CAN be done! (Abstract). *ASHA Leader, 7*(15), 96. (Seminar presented at the Annual Convention of the American Speech-Language-Hearing Association, Atlanta, GA.)

Riley, G. (1994). *Stuttering severity instrument for children and adults* (3rd ed.). Austin, TX: Pro-Ed.

Riley, G. & Costello Ingham, J. (2000). Acoustic duration changes associated with two types of treatment for children who stutter. *Journal of Speech and Hearing Research, 43*, 965-978.

Riley, G. & Riley, J. (1985). *Oral-motor assessment and treatment: Improving syllable production.* Austin, TX: Pro-Ed.

Riley, G. & Riley, J. (1986). Oral-motor discoordination among children who stutter. *Journal of Fluency Disorders, 11*, 335-334.

Ryan, B. (1974). *Programmed therapy for stuttering in children and adults.* Springfield, IL: Charles C. Thomas.

Shapiro, D. (1999). *Stuttering Intervention: A collaborative journey to fluency freedom.* Austin, TX: Pro-Ed.

Sheehan, J.G. (1970). *Stuttering: Research and Therapy.* New York: Harper & Row.

Sheehan, J.G. (1975). Conflict theory and avoidance-reduction therapy. In J. Eisenson (Ed.), *Stuttering: A second symposium* (pp. 97-198). New York: Harper & Row.

Silverman, F.H. (1996). *Stuttering and other fluency disorders.* Needham Heights, MA: Allyn & Bacon.

Sisskin, V. (2002). Therapy planning for school-age children who stutter. *Seminars in Speech and Language, 23*, 173-179.

Smith, A. & Kelly, E.M. (1997). Stuttering: A dynamic, multifactorial model. In R. Curlee & G. Siegel (Eds.), *Nature and treatment of stuttering: New directions.* (2nd ed., pp. 204-217). Needham Heights, MA: Allyn & Bacon.

St. Louis, K. & Hinzman, A. (1988). A descriptive study of speech, language, and hearing characteristics of school-age stutterers. *Journal of Fluency Disorders, 13*, 331-355.

St. Louis, K. & Westbrook, J. (1987). The effectiveness of treatment for stuttering. In L. Rustin, D. Rowley, & H. Purser (Eds.), *Progress in the treatment of fluency disorders* (pp. 235-257). London: Taylor and Francis.

St. Louis, K.O. (1999). Person-first labeling and stuttering. *Journal of Fluency Disorders, 24*, 1-24.

St. Louis, K.O. & Durrenberger, C.H. (1993). What communication disorders do experienced clinicians prefer to manage? *Asha, 35*, 23-31.

Starkweather, C.W. & Givens-Ackerman, J. (1997). *Stuttering.* Austin, TX: Pro-Ed.

Susca, M., Scott Trautman, L., & Healey, E.C. (2002). *A multidimensional rating scale for characterizing children who stutter.* Annual meeting of the American Speech-Language-Hearing Association, Atlanta, GA.

Tellis, G. & Tellis, C. (2003). Multicultural issues in school settings. *Seminars in Speech and Language, 24*, 21-26.

Throneburg, R. & Yairi, E. (1994). Temporal dynamics of repetitions during the early stage of childhood stuttering: an acoustic study. *Journal of Speech and Hearing Research. 37*, 1067-1075.

Van Borsel, J., Maes, E., & Foulon, S. (2001). Stuttering and bilingualism: A review. *Journal of Fluency Disorders, 26*, 179-205.

Van Riper, C. (1973). *Treatment of stuttering.* New Jersey: Prentice Hall.

Van Riper, C. (1982). *The nature of stuttering* (2nd ed.). Englewood Cliffs, NJ: Prentice-Hall.

Williams, D.E. (1957). A point of view about "stuttering." *Journal of Speech and Hearing Disorders, 22*, 3, 390-397.

Williams, D.E. (1971). Stuttering therapy for children. In L.E. Travis (Ed.), *Handbook of Speech Pathology and Audiology.* New York: Appleton-Century-Crofts.

Williams, D.E. (1979). A perspective on approaches to stuttering therapy. In Gregory, H.H. (Ed.). *Controversies about stuttering therapy.* Baltimore: University Park Press.

Williams, D. & Dugan, P. (2002). Administering stuttering modification therapy in school settings. *Seminars in Speech and Language, 23*, 187-194.

Wolk, L., Edwards, M.L., & Conture, E.G. (1993). Coexistence of stuttering and disordered phonology in young children. *Journal of Speech and Hearing Research, 36*, 906-917.

Wolpe, J. (1958). *Psychotherapy by reciprocal inhibition.* Stanford, CA.: Stanford University Press.

Yairi, E. (1996). Applications of disfluencies in measurements of stuttering. *Journal of Speech and Hearing Research, 39*, 402-404.

Yairi, E. (1997). Disfluency characteristics of childhood stuttering. In R.F. Curlee & G.M. Siegel (Eds.), *Nature and treatment of stuttering: New directions* (2nd ed.). Boston: Allyn and Bacon.

Yairi E. & Ambrose N. (1999). Early childhood stuttering I: Persistency and recovery rates. *Journal of Speech and Hearing Research. 42*, 1097-112.

Yairi, E., Ambrose, N., Paden, E.P., & Throneburg, R.N. (1996). Predictive factors of persistence and recovery: Pathways of childhood stuttering. *Journal of Communication Disorders, 29,* 51-77.

Yairi, E. & Lewis, B. (1984). Disfluencies at the onset of stuttering. *Journal of Speech and Hearing Research, 27,* 154-159.

Yaruss, J.S. (1997a). Clinical implications of situational variability in preschool children who stutter. *Journal of Fluency Disorders, 22,* 187-203.

Yaruss, J.S. (1997b). Clinical measurement of stuttering behaviors. *Contemporary Issues in Communication Science and Disorders, 24,* 33-44.

Yaruss, J.S. (1998a). Describing the consequences of disorders: Stuttering and the International Classification of Impairments, Disabilities, and Handicaps. *Journal of Speech and Hearing Research, 49,* 249-257.

Yaruss, J.S. (1998b). Real-time analysis of speech fluency: Procedures and reliability training. *American Journal of Speech-Language Pathology, 7(2),* 25-37.

Yaruss, J.S. (1998c). Treatment outcomes in stuttering: Finding value in clinical data. In A. Cordes & R. Ingham (Eds.), *Toward treatment efficacy in stuttering: A search for empirical bases* (pp. 213-242). Austin, TX: Pro-Ed.

Yaruss, J.S. (2000). Converting between word and syllable counts in children's conversational speech samples. *Journal of Fluency Disorders, 25,* 305-316.

Yaruss, J.S. (Ed.) (2002). Facing the Challenge of Treating Stuttering in the Schools (Part I: Selecting Goals and Strategies for Success). *Seminars in Speech and Language, 23,* 3. (First of two issues of *Seminars* focused on treating stuttering in school-age children.)

Yaruss, J.S. (Ed.) (2003). Facing the Challenge of Treating Stuttering in the Schools (Part II: One Size Does Not Fit All). *Seminars in Speech and Language, 24,* 1. (Second of two issues of *Seminars* focused on treating stuttering in school-age children.)

Yaruss, J.S., LaSalle, L.R., & Conture, E.G. (1998). Evaluating stuttering in young children: Diagnostic data. *American Journal of Speech-Language Pathology, 7(4),* 62-76.

Yaruss, J.S., Max, M., Newman, R., & Campbell, J. (1998). Comparing real-time and transcript-based techniques for measuring stuttering. *Journal of Fluency Disorders, 23,* 137-151.

Yaruss, J.S. & Quesal, R.W. (2002). Research Based Stuttering Therapy Revisited. *Perspectives on Fluency and Fluency Disorders, 12(2),* 22-24.

Yaruss, J.S., Quesal, R.W., Reeves, L., Molt, L., Kluetz, B., Caruso, A.J., Lewis, F., & McClure, J.A. (2002). Speech treatment and support group experiences of people who participate in the National Stuttering Association. *Journal of Fluency Disorders, 27,* 115-135.

Yaruss, J.S. & Reardon, N.A. (2002a). Successful communication for children who stutter: Finding the balance. *Seminars in Speech and Language, 23,* 195-204.

Yaruss, J. S. & Reardon, N. (2002b). *Preschool children who stutter: Information and support for parents* (2nd ed.). Anaheim Hills, CA: National Stuttering Association.

Yaruss, J.S. & Reardon, N.A., (2003). Fostering generalization and maintenance in school settings. *Seminars in Speech and Language, 24,* 33-40.

Zebrowski, P.M. (1991). Duration of the speech disfluencies of beginning stutterers. *Journal of Speech and Hearing Research, 34,* 481-491.

Zebrowski, P.M. (1994). Duration of sound prolongation and sound/syllable repetition in children who stutter: Preliminary observations. *Journal of Speech and Hearing Research, 37,* 254-263.

Zebrowski, P.M. (1997). Assisting young children who stutter and their families: Defining the role of the speech-language pathologist. *American Journal of Speech-Language Pathology, 6(2),* 19-28.

Zebrowski, P. & Cilek, T. (1997). Stuttering therapy in the elementary school setting: Guidelines for clinician-teacher collaboration. *Seminars in Speech and Language, 18,* 329-340.

Zebrowski, P.M. & Conture, E.G. (1997). Influence of nontreatment variables on treatment effectiveness for school-age children who stutter. In A.K. Cordes & R.J. Ingham (Eds.), *Treatment efficacy for stuttering: A search for empirical bases,* (pp. 293-310). San Diego: Singular Publishing.

Zebrowski, P.M. & Schum, R.L. (1993). Counseling parents of children who stutter. *American Journal of Speech-Language Pathology, 2,* 65-73.

21-03-987654321